Handbook of Enteral, Parenteral, and ARC/AIDS Nutritional Therapy

P9-CDY-307

Handbook of Enteral, Parenteral, and ARC/AIDS Nutritional Therapy

MICHAEL S. HICKEY, M.D.
Assistant Clinical Professor of Surgery
University of California at San Francisco
Surgical Director, Nutrition Support Service
San Francisco General Hospital
San Francisco, California

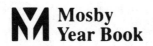

Mosby Year Book

St. Louis   Baltimore   Boston   Chicago   London   Philadelphia   Sydney   Toronto

▼▼ Mosby
Year Book

Dedicated to Publishing Excellence

Sponsoring Editor: Dana Dreibelbis
Developmental Editor: Ellen Thomas
Associate Managing Editor, Manuscript Services: Deborah Thorp
Production Manager: Nancy C. Baker
Proofroom Manager: Barbara Kelly

Copyright © 1992 by Mosby–Year Book, Inc.
A C. V. Mosby Company imprint of Mosby–Year Book, Inc.

Mosby–Year Book, Inc.
11830 Westline Industrial Drive
St. Louis, MO 63146

All rights reserved. No part of this publication may be reproduced, stored in a retrieval system, or transmitted, in any form or by any means, electronic, mechanical, photocopying, recording, or otherwise, without prior written permission from the publisher. Printed in the United States of America.

Permission to photocopy or reproduce solely for internal or personal use is permitted for libraries or other users registered with the Copyright Clearance Center, provided that the base fee of $4.00 per chapter plus $.10 per page is paid directly to the Copyright Clearance Center, 21 Congress Street, Salem, MA 01970. This consent does not extend to other kinds of copying, such as copying for general distribution, for advertising or promotional purposes, for creating new collected works, or for resale.

1 2 3 4 5 6 7 8 9 0 CL/ML 96 95 94 93 92

Library of Congress Cataloging-in-Publication Data
Hickey, Michael S.
   Handbook of enteral, parenteral, and ARC/AIDS nutritional therapy
/ Michael S. Hickey.
     p. cm.
   Includes index.
   ISBN 1-55664-341-1
   1. Enteral feeding—Handbooks, manuals, etc. 2. Parenteral
feeding—Handbooks, manuals, etc. 3. AIDS (Disease)—Diet therapy—
-Handbooks, manuals, etc. I. Title.
   [DNLM: 1. Acquired Immunodeficiency Syndrome—diet therapy.
2. AIDS-Related Complex—diet therapy. 3. Enteral Feeding.
4. Nutritional Status. 5. Parenteral Feeding. WD 308 H628h]
RM225.H53 1991
615.8′55—dc20   91-31227
DNLM/DLC   CIP
for Library of Congress

I wish to dedicate this manual to my father, Robert Hickey, and my two daughters, Allison and Michelle Hickey. Thank you for all your support and encouragement during the writing of this text.

PREFACE

Nutrition plays a key role in the successful management of critically ill patients. During the past decade, there have been significant advances in the field of nutritional therapy. Nutritionists no longer have a limited therapeutic arsenal. Instead, they now have precise methods for calculating the patient's energy requirement per indirect calorimetry; specialized amino acid, polypeptide, and immune-regulating enteral diets for patients with compromised gut function; specific amino acid parenteral diets for fluid-restricted and both renal and hepatic failure patients; and new synthetic hormones for enhancing protein assimilation and controlling diarrhea. Because of these advances, the development of new therapeutic regimens, and exciting new research, nutrition continues to be an interesting, integral aspect of patient care.

Physicians, nurses, dietitians, and pharmacists have a basic knowledge of nutritional therapy. Because of either their specialty interests or practice commitments, they rarely have an opportunity to attend formal nutrition conferences. Consequently, they are unaware of the new advances in this field. Although they have a strong desire to expand their knowledge, time constraints and other commitments prohibit their continuing education in this area.

This manual was written to provide practicing physicians, nurses, dietitians, and medical students with both basic and new information regarding nutritional assessment, enteral and parenteral diet therapy, and the nutritional management of ARC and AIDS patients. It discusses the important aspects of nutritional therapy in a straightforward, simplified manner. Self-assessment questions are provided for each chapter to facilitate the reader's review of salient points discussed in the text.

The manual will simplify the delivery of safe, efficacious, appropriate nutritional therapy. The primary goal of this text is to advance the knowledge of medical personnel about nutritional therapy and, ultimately, to improve patient care.

Michael S. Hickey, M.D.

CONTENTS

NUTRITIONAL ASSESSMENT GUIDELINES

1

GENERAL DISCUSSION

Clinicians clearly recognize the role of nutrition in the successful management of critically ill patients. Nutrition studies have revealed that nearly 50% of all hospitalized surgical and medical patients would benefit from some form of nutritional supplementation.* A normal, well-balanced diet provides 1 g of protein per kilogram of body weight daily. The daily intake of 10 g of nitrogen or 62.5 g of protein (1 g nitrogen = 6.25 g protein) promotes positive nitrogen balance and prevents protein malnutrition in most adults. The body can assimilate a maximum of 10 g of protein per kilogram body weight daily. This amounts to nearly 700 g of protein or more than 100 g of nitrogen in the average 70-kg adult. Adult daily caloric requirements are dependent on the clinical situation. During the hypermetabolic phase (HMP) of acute injury or illness, patients can successfully metabolize a maximum of 30 to 35 kcal/kg.[124] However, following the HMP, they can assimilate as much as 35 to 45 kcal/kg.†

TYPES OF MALNUTRITION

Patients with inadequate nutrient intake may become malnourished. There are basically two types of malnutrition: (1) protein malnutrition, which occurs when the diet is deficient in protein, and (2) protein-calorie malnutrition, which occurs when the diet is deficient in both protein and calories.

---

*References 10, 11, 30, 46, 84, 114, 123, 124.
†References 39, 71, 82, 83, 90, 97, 121, 122.

Protein Malnutrition (Kwashiorkor Syndrome)

Protein malnutrition results in

- Muscle atrophy
- Delayed wound healing[99]
- Prolonged ventilatory dependence
- Impaired immunocompetence[9, 20, 26]
- Delayed bone callus formation
- Abnormal red cell function.

Protein malnutrition may occur as a result of inadequate protein intake, chronic diarrhea, renal dysfunction, infection,[119] hemorrhage, trauma, burns, or critical illness. It is characterized by

- Reduced serum albumin and transferrin levels[65, 103]
- Decreased serum iron-binding capacity
- Delayed cellular immunity.[9, 20, 26, 49, 50]

The weight loss that occurs with protein malnutrition is inconsistent and may not be recognized because of fluid retention. The clinical and chemical findings that occur in patients with protein malnutrition are described as the kwashiorkor syndrome.

The protein losses that occur during critical illness are primarily the result of protein tissue catabolism. These losses are determined by measuring the 24-hour urinary urea nitrogen (UUN) excretion[35, 52] (Table 1–1). Most body proteins contain 16% protein. By dividing 16 into 100, a constant (6.25) is derived. By multiplying 6.25 times the total urinary nitrogen loss, one can calculate the total protein loss. To determine the equivalent amount of catabolized lean wet tissue such as muscle, it is necessary to multiply 6.25×5 because muscle protein is bound to 4 volumes of water by weight. Thus, 1 g of urinary nitrogen represents the catabolism of approximately 30 g of muscle tissue. An even more precise method for determining the degree of skeletal muscle catabolism involves measuring the 24-hour urinary excretion of 3-methyl histidine, a nonreducible product of skeletal muscle degradation.[36, 75, 95]

In addition to protein losses secondary to catabolism, patients may have direct intact protein losses. Whole blood contains approximately 3 g nitrogen or 19 g of protein/100 mL of blood. Consequently, significant hemorrhage may result in major plasma protein losses. Pneumonia and empyema result in intrathoracic plasma protein losses. Intestinal obstruction and peritonitis result

TABLE 1–1.

24-Hour Nitrogen Balance Determination

Nitrogen balance = $[Nitrogen]^{(intake)} - [Nitrogen]^{(output)}$

$$[Nitrogen]^{(intake)} = \left[\frac{g\ protein}{6.25\ g\ Protein/g\ nitrogen} \right]$$

$$[Nitrogen]^{(output)} = \left[UUN^* \times \frac{1,000\ mL}{L} \times 24\text{-Hr urine volume (L)} \times \frac{g\ Nitrogen}{1,000\ mg\ Nitrogen} + 3 \right]$$

$$^*UUN = \frac{mg\ nitrogen}{100\ mL\ urine}$$

in significant losses of plasma protein into the bowel wall and the peritoneal space. Crush injuries and thermal injuries give rise to soft tissue and burn wound protein losses.

Protein-Calorie Malnutrition (Marasmus Syndrome)

Protein-calorie malnutrition occurs as a result of inadequate nutrient intake (protein and calories). This condition results in

- Bradycardia
- Hypothermia
- Reduced basal metabolism
- Depletion of subcutaneous fat and tissue turgor
- Development of wrinkled skin.[9, 12, 20, 26, 34, 49, 66, 71]

Patients with protein-calorie malnutrition, in contrast to those with protein malnutrition, consistently lose weight. The clinical and chemical findings that occur in patients with protein-calorie malnutrition are described as the marasmus syndrome.

POTENTIAL ENERGY SOURCES
Mechanisms for Avoiding Malnutrition During Periods of Metabolic Stress

The body's ability to avoid malnutrition during periods of metabolic stress is dependent on its

1. Utilization of endogenous energy stores and available biochemically active substrates.
2. Assimilation of exogenous calories and protein.
3. Successful mobilization of energy stores.[105]

Three Sources Of Energy

The body has three potential energy sources: carbohydrate (glycogen), protein, and fat (triglycerides).

Glycogen

Glycogen is combined with water and is stored in both the muscle (120 to 130 g) and the liver (60 to 70 g). Glycogen metabolism yields only 2 kcal/g, in contrast to carbohydrate metabolism which yields 4 kcal/g. The body's entire glycogen reserve is consumed after 18 to 24 hours of complete starvation.

Protein

Protein is stored primarily in muscle. The metabolism of muscle protein yields 2 kcal/g. Body proteins are not designed as a primary fuel source; instead, they function as organic catalysts (enzymes), cellular building blocks, antibodies, and hormones. Protein that is not utilized to replenish body stores is metabolized and then excreted as urea nitrogen. Excess calories produced from protein metabolism are stored as fat.

Fat

Fat is essentially water free and yields approximately 9 kcal/g. Fat catabolism provides 87% of caloric requirements during periods of metabolic stress and starvation.

Metabolic Events That Occur During Starvation in a 70-kg Individual

Studies have demonstrated that the following metabolic events occur if a 70-kg man who consumes approximately 1,800 kcal daily is subjected to a 24-hour period of starvation:

1. The body catabolizes 75 g of protein (primarily from muscle) and 160 g of triglyceride from adipose tissue.
2. The body excretes 12 to 15 g of urinary nitrogen, primarily in the form of urea.
3. The total body weight decreases approximately 500 g.
4. Body glycogen stores yield approximately 180 g of endogenous glucose for ongoing metabolism.
5. The body derives 87% of its caloric requirements from fat and 13% from protein tissue catabolism.

The body composition of a healthy 70-kg man and the calories derived from each potential fuel source are listed in Table 1–2.

TABLE 1–2.

Body Composition of a Healthy 70-kg Adult Man

Weight (kg)	Components	Calories Equivalent
46.7	Water and minerals	0
15.0	Fat (adipose triglyceride)	141.000
6.0	Protein (mainly muscle)	24.000
	Glycogen	
0.190	Muscle	600
0.075	Liver	300
69.925*		165.900*
0.020	Glucose (extracellular fluid)	80
0.0003	Free fatty acids (plasma)	3
0.003	Triglycerides (plasma)	30
69.9483†		166.013†

Adapted from Cahill GF. *N Engl J Med* 1970; 282.
*Subtotal.
†Total.

NUTRITIONAL ASSESSMENT

A nutritional assessment includes (1) an evaluation of the key nutritional indices: protein (visceral and somatic) and fat reserves,* (2) a 24-hour nitrogen balance determination,[35, 52] (3) assessment of gastrointestinal function and (4) a determination of the daily caloric and protein requirements.[39, 67, 73, 74, 97, 121, 122]

Evaluation of Protein (Visceral and Somatic) and Fat Reserves

The visceral protein reserve is estimated from the serum total protein, albumin, and transferrin levels; total lymphocyte count; and antigen skin testing. The somatic (skeletal) protein reserve is evaluated by determining the creatinine/height index. The fat reserve is assessed per anthropometric measurement of the biceps and triceps skinfold or electrical impedance studies. Of all three indices, the visceral protein reserve is considered the most important index of nutritional status. Table 1–3 is a list of the normal values for each of these indices; abnormal values are categorized

*References 3, 4, 13, 15, 31, 42, 46, 47, 59, 77, 82.

TABLE 1–3.

Assessment of Protein and Fat Reserves

Clinical/Laboratory Parameters	Extent of Malnutrition		
	Mild	Moderate*	Severe*
Albumin, (g/dL)†	2.8–3.2	2.1–2.7	<2.1
Transferrin, (mg/dL)†	150–200	100–150	<100
Total lymphocyte count (cells/mm³)†	1,200–2,000	800–1,200	<800
Creatinine/height index (%) (actual/ideal × 100)‡	60–80	40–60	<40
Ideal body weight (%)	80–90	70–80	<70
Usual body weight, (%)	85–95	75–85	<75
Weight loss/unit time	<5%/mo	<2%/wk	>2%/wk
	<7.5%/3 mo	>5%/mo	
	<10%/6 mo	>7.5%/3 mo	
		>10%/6 mo	
Skin tests (no. reactive/no. placed)	4/4 (normal)	1–2/4 (weak)	0/0 (anergic)

Normal anthropometric measurements	Male		Female
Triceps skinfold, (mm)§	12.5		16.5
Mid-arm circumference, (cm)	29.3		28.5

*Nutritional therapy indicated.
†Visceral protein reserve.
‡Somatic protein reserve.
§Fat reserve.

in terms of mild, moderate, and severe malnutrition. Nutritional therapy is indicated when these indices suggest either moderate or severe malnutrition.†

Nitrogen Balance Determination

A nitrogen balance determination is very helpful in assessing the pretreatment nutritional status and monitoring the response to nutritional therapy. All critically ill patients should undergo a weekly nitrogen balance determination while receiving enteral or parenteral nutritional therapy. It is performed by collecting a 24-hour urine specimen for urinary urea nitrogen and then determining the actual urinary nitrogen loss (nitrogen output). This value is

†References 3, 4, 13, 15, 31, 42, 46, 47, 59, 77, 82.

subsequently subtracted from the nitrogen intake to determine the 24-hour nitrogen balance[35, 52] (Table 1–1). A precise nitrogen balance determination should also include gastrointestinal nitrogen losses.

Patients in positive nitrogen balance usually do not require aggressive nutritional therapy. In contrast, patients in negative nitrogen balance should receive aggressive nutritional therapy.

Assessment of Gastrointestinal Function

Gastrointestinal function must be considered during the initial nutritional assessment. Critically ill medical, surgical, and trauma patients with normal or minimal gut dysfunction and normal pre-illness nutritional indices who will probably resume adequate oral food intake in less than 7 days do not routinely require nutritional therapy. In contrast, patients with either (1) abnormal pre-illness nutritional indices *or* (2) severe gut dysfunction which predictably will not improve in 5 to 7 days will require aggressive enteral or parenteral nutritional therapy.

TABLE 1–4.
Adult Nonburn Daily Caloric and Protein Requirements

Estimate:

Calories (total kcal)

Male/female: 25–30/kg (weight loss)
25–35/kg (weight maintenance) → 30–35/kg (weight maintenance)
35–40/kg (weight gain)

Protein (gm)

Male/female: 0.8–2.0/kg

Calculate:

Calories (total kcal) for weight maintenance

Male = $[66.5 + (13.7 \times \text{wt kg}) + (5 \times \text{ht cm}) - (6.7 \times \text{age yr})] \times \text{AF}^* \times \text{IF}\dagger$

Female = $[665.1 + (9.6 \times \text{wt kg}) + (1.8 \times \text{ht cm}) - (4.7 \times \text{age yr})] \times \text{AF}^* \times \text{IF}\dagger$

Note: Add 500 kcal to the equations above for weight gain

Protein (g)

Male/female = $\text{Total kcal} \times \dfrac{\text{g Nitrogen}}{150 \text{ kcal}} \times \dfrac{6.25 \text{ g Protein}}{\text{g Nitrogen}}$

Activity factor:		†*Injury factor:*	
Confined to bed	1.2	Surgery	1.1–1.2
Ambulatory	1.3	Infection	1.2–1.6
Fever factor	1.13/°C > 37° C	Trauma	1.1–1.8
		Sepsis	1.4–1.8

Determination of Daily Caloric and Protein Requirements

Prior to initiating nutritional therapy, the patient's daily caloric and protein requirements are estimated and a nutritional regimen designed. Daily caloric and protein requirements are dependent on the clinical situation.

Adult Nonburn Requirements

Adult nonburn daily caloric and protein requirements may be estimated or calculated (Table 1–4) or determined per indirect calorimetry (IC), which is most accurate.* Calculation affords a more accurate determination of the patient's nutritional requirements, and is preferable to estimating the requirements. The equation used to calculate the adult (nonburn) daily caloric requirement is derived from a combination of both the Harris-Benedict equation and specific activity and injury factors. The adult daily protein requirement usually ranges from 0.8 to 2.0 g/kg. It may, however, be substantially greater than 2.0 g/kg depending upon the patient's pre-injury protein status and the specific clinical situation.

Adult Burn Requirements

Adult burn (>20% total body surface area) daily caloric and protein requirements are calculated by using a modified version of the Curreri formula (Table 1–5) or determined per IC.*

Requirements for Adult AIDS and ARC Patients

The daily caloric and protein requirements for adult patients suffering from the autoimmune deficiency syndrome (AIDS) or AIDS-related complex (ARC) are either estimated or calculated (Table 1–6) or determined per IC. Calculation affords a more accurate determination of the patient's nutritional requirements. Hence, it is preferable to estimating the requirement. The equation used to calculate their caloric requirements is derived from a combination of the Harris-Benedict equation and specific activity and injury factors plus the addition of 500 to 1,000 kcal.

Pediatric Nonburn Requirements

Pediatric nonburn daily caloric and protein requirements are age and weight dependent. Table 1–7 lists the caloric and protein requirements of pediatric patients based on their age and weight. Pediatric patients 15 years of age and older have the same caloric and protein requirements as the adult nonburn patient (see Table 1–4).

*References 39, 73, 74, 97, 119, 121, 122, 124.

TABLE 1-5.

Adult Burn (>20% TBSA*) Daily Caloric and Protein Requirements

---

Estimate:

Calories (total kcal)

Male/female: Maintenance + 40 kcal/% TBSA* burn

Protein (gm)

Male/female: 1.5–2.5/kg

Calculate:

Calories (total kcal) for weight maintenance

Male = (25 kcal × preburn wt kg × BMR† age factor) + (40 kcal × % TBSA burn)

Female = (22 kcal × preburn wt kg × BMR age factor) + (40 kcal × % TBSA burn)

Note: Add 500 kcal to the equations above for weight gain

Protein (g)

Male/female = (1 g protein × preburn wt kg) + (3 × % TBSA burn)

---

*TBSA = total body surface area.

†BMR = basal metabolic rate: 20–40 yr = 1.00
40–50 yr = 0.95
50–75 yr = 0.90
>75 yr = 0.80

TABLE 1-6.

Adult ARC and AIDS Daily Caloric and Protein Requirements

Estimate:

Calories (total kcal)

Male/female: 35–40/kg

Protein (g)

Male/female: 2.0–2.5/kg

Calculate:

Calories (total kcal) for weight maintenance

Male = [66.5 + (13.7 × wt kg) + (5 × ht cm) − (6.7 × age yr)] × AF* × IF† + 500 kcal

Female = [665.1 + (9.6 × wt kg) + (1.8 × ht cm) − (4.7 × age yr)] × AF* × IF† + 500 kcal

Note: Add 500 kcal to the equations above for weight gain

Protein (g)

$$\text{Male/female} = \text{Total kcal} \times \frac{\text{g nitrogen}}{150 \text{ kcal}} \times \frac{6.25 \text{ g protein}}{\text{g nitrogen}}$$

---

*Activity factor		†Injury factor	
Confined to bed	1.2	Surgery	1.1–1.2
Ambulatory	1.3	Infection	1.2–1.6
Fever factor	1.13/°C > 37° C.	Trauma	1.1–1.8
		Sepsis	1.4–1.8.

TABLE 1-7.

Pediatric Nonburn Daily Caloric and Protein Requirements

Age	kcal/kg	Protein, g/kg
Newborn term	117	1.8
Newborn premature	130	1.8
3 days term	130	2.2
3 days premature	130	2.2
10 days	130	2.2
3 mo	100-130	3.5-4.0
6 mo	100-130	3.5-4.0
9 mo	100-130	3.5
1-3 yr	90-100	2.5
4-6 yr	80-90	2.2
7-9 yr	70-80	2.2
10-12 yr	60-70	1.8
13-15 yr	50-60	1.7
15+ yr	40-50	1.4

Diets should provide 100-125 nonprotein carbohydrate calories per gram nitrogen administered..

(*Note:* **1 g nitrogen = 6.25 g protein**).

Pediatric Burn Requirements

Pediatric burn (<10% total body surface area) daily caloric and protein requirements are calculated by using a modified version of the Curreri formula (Table 1-8).*

Indications for Nutritional Therapy

Nutritional therapy is indicated if the nutritional assessment reveals one or more of the values listed in Table 1-9. The general criteria for starting nutritional therapy are as follows:

Nutritional Status	Nutrional Management
Clinically well-nourished, preinjury serum albumin >2.5 g/dL, and oral diet anticipated <7 days	Observe for 7 days; if oral feedings *not* tolerated, begin special enteral or parenteral diet
Clinically well-nourished, preinjury serum albumin >2.5 g/dL and oral diet *not* anticipated <7 days	Begin special enteral or parenteral diet within 72 hr
Clinically malnourished, preinjury serum albumin <2.5 g/dL, and metabolically stressed	Begin special enteral or parenteral diet within 72 hr

*References 8, 28, 29, 45, 57, 81, 90, 100, 104, 106, 107, 109, 116.

TABLE 1–8.

Pediatric Burn (>10% TBSA*) Daily Caloric and Protein Requirements

	Maintenance Caloric Requirements		
Age	kcal/kg	Age	kcal/kg
Newborn term	117	9 mo	100–130
Newborn premature	130	1–3 yr	90–100
3 days term	130	4–6 yr	80–90
3 days premature	130	7–9 yr	70–80
10 days	130	10–12 yr	60–70
3 mo	100–130	13–15 yr	50–60
6 mo	100–130	15+ yr	40–50

Estimate:
  Calories (total kcal)
    Male/female: Maintenance calories + 40 kcal/% TBSA* burn
  Protein (g)
    Male/female: 1.4–4.0/kg
Calculate:
  Calories (total kcal) for weight maintenance
    Male   = Maintenance calories + 40 kcal/% TBSA burn
    Female = Maintenance calories + 40 kcal/% TBSA burn
    Note: Add 500 kcal to the equations above for weight gain
  Protein (gm)
    Male/female = (1 g protein × preburn wt kg) + (3 × % TBSA burn)

*TBSA = total body surface area.

TABLE 1–9.

Indications for Nutritional Therapy

Nutritional Indices	Value
Total protein, (g/dL)	<6.0
Albumin, (g/dL)	<2.7
Transferrin, (mg/dL)	<150
Total lymphocyte count (cells/hpf)	<1,200
Antigen skin test, (no. reactive/no. placed)	2/4
Creatinine/height index, (%)	<60
Triceps skin fold, (mm)	<12.5 (female)
	<16.5 (male)
Nitrogen balance	Negative or zero

TABLE 1–10.

Adult Daily Requirements of Electrolytes, Trace Metals, Vitamins, and Minerals

Substance	Enteral	Parenteral
Electrolyte		
Sodium	90–150 mEq	90–150 mEq
Potassium	60–90 mEq	60–90 mEq
Trace metal		
Chromium*·†	5–200 µg	10–15 µg
Copper*·†	2–3 mg	0.5–0.15 mg
Manganese*·†	2.5–5.0 mg	0.15–0.8 mg
Zinc*	15 mg	2.5–4.0 mg
Iron	10 mg	2.5 mg
Iodine	150 µg	—
Fluoride†	1.5–4.0 mg	—
Selenium†	0.05–0.20 mg	20–40 µg
Molybdenum†	0.15–0.50 mg	20–120 µg
Tin‡	—	—
Vanadium‡	—	—
Nickel‡	—	—
Arsenic‡	—	—
Silicon‡	—	—
Vitamin		
Ascorbic acid (C)§	60 mg	100 mg
Retinol (A)§	1,000 µg	3,300 IU
Vitamin D§	5.0 µg	200 IU
Thiamine (B_1)	1.4 mg	3.0 mg
Riboflavin (B_2)§	1.7 mg	3.6 mg
Pyridoxine (B_6)§	2.2 mg	4.0 mg
Niacin§	19 mg	40 mg
Pantothenic acid§	4–7 mg	15 mg
Vitamin E§	10.0 mg	10 IU
Biotin†·§	100–200 µg	60 µg
Folic acid§	400 µg	400 µg
Cobalamin (B_{12})§	3.0 µg	5.0 µg
Vitamin K‖	70–140 µg	10 mg
Mineral		
Calcium	800 mg	0.20–0.30 mEq/kg
Phosphorus	800 mg	300–400 mg/kg
Magnesium	350 mg	0.34–0.45 mEq/kg
Sulfur	2–3 g	—

*Multitrace brand, 5 mL, provides the normal daily requirement.
†Estimated safe and adequate dose.
‡No data available regarding human requirements.
§MVI-12, 10 mL, provides the normal daily requirement.
‖Weekly requirement.

TABLE 1–11.

Pediatric Daily Fluid Requirements

Weight (kg)	Fluid
0–10	100 cc/kg
10–20	1,000 cc + (50 cc/kg for every kg >10 but <20)
20–30	1,500 ml + (20 cc/kg for every kg >20 but <30)
>30	2,000–2,500 cc

SELECTION OF A NUTRITIONAL THERAPY REGIMEN

The selection of a nutritional therapy regimen requires the consideration of several factors. The diet should deliver 75 to 150 nonprotein carbohydrate calories per gram of nitrogen administered. It should also provide the patient's daily required

- Calories and protein (see Tables 1–4 to 1–8)
- Fat
- Electrolytes, trace metals, vitamins, and minerals (Table 1–10)
- Fluids.

The volume of the enteral or parenteral diet administered should not exceed the patient's daily fluid requirement. Therefore, prior to selecting an enteral diet or formulating a parenteral diet, a clinician must accurately determine the patient's daily fluid requirement. The daily maintenance fluid requirement for an adult 70-kg patient ranges from 2,000 to 2,500 cc. The pediatric daily maintenance fluid requirement is weight dependent (Table 1–11).

In addition to the maintenance fluid requirement, one must also consider the fluid losses that occur secondary to nasogastric drainage, fistulae, diarrhea, and febrile episodes (10% increase in the maintenance fluid requirement for every degree increase in temperature above 37° C). Patients with significant nasogastric or fistula drainage or diarrhea may have fluctuations in their serum electrolytes and acid-base balance. Enteral and parenteral diets should replace these gastrointestinal tract electrolyte and bicarbonate losses. The electrolyte and bicarbonate composition of several of the key gastrointestinal secretions are listed in Table 1–12.

MONITORING THERAPEUTIC RESPONSE
Monitoring Schedules for Enteral and Parenteral Diet Therapy

Patients undergoing nutritional therapy must be monitored closely. The specific therapeutic monitoring schedule is dependent

TABLE 1-12.

Electrolyte and Bicarbonate Composition of Gastrointestinal Secretions

Type of Secretion	Volume (cc/24 hr)	Na (mEq/L)	K (mEq/L)	Cl (mEq/L)	HCO₃ (mEq/L)
Saliva	1,500	10	26	10	30
	(500–2000)	(2–10)	(20–30)	(8–18)	—
Stomach	1,500	60	10	130	—
	(100–4000)	(9–116)	(0–32)	(8–154)	—
Duodenum	—	140	5	80	—
	(100–2,000)	—	—	—	—
Ileum	3,000	140	5	104	30
	(100–9000)	(80–150)	(2–8)	(43–137)	—
Colon	—	60	30	40	—
Bile	—	145	5	100	35
	(50–800)	(131–164)	(3–12)	(89–180)	—
Pancreas	—	140	5	75	115
	(100–800)	(113–185)	(3–7)	(54–95)	—

TABLE 1-13.

Monitoring Schedules for Enteral and Parenteral Diet Therapy

Enteral therapy

Monday A.M.	Begin a 24-hr urine collection for urinary urea nitrogen (UUN) to determine the patient's nitrogen balance
Thursday A.M.	CBC, SMAC-20, copper, zinc, magnesium, transferrin, triglyceride, prealbumin, and retinol binding protein
Daily	Weight (kg)
Weekly	Nutritional assessment

Parenteral therapy

Sunday A.M.	CBC and SMAC-20
Monday A.M.	Begin a 24-hr urine collection for UUN to determine the patient's nitrogen balance
Tuesday A.M.	Electrolytes, BUN, creatinine and glucose
Thursday A.M.	CBC, SMAC-20, copper, zinc, magnesium, transferrin, triglyceride, prealbumin, and retinol binding protein
Daily	Weight (kg)
Weekly	Nutritional assessment

on the nutritional therapy regimen administered. The recommended monitoring schedules for both enteral and parenteral diet therapy are shown in Table 1–13.

REFERENCES

1. Abbott WC, et al: Nutritional care of the trauma patient. *Surg Gynecol Obstet* 1983; 150:585–597.

2. Askanazi J, et al: Nutrition for the patient with respiratory failure: Glucose vs. fat. *Anesthesiology* 1981; 54:373–377.

3. Baker JP, et al: Nutritional assessment: A comparison of clinical judgment and objective measures. *N Engl J Med* 1982; 306:969–972.

4. Barker BC, Weaver KE, Hickey MS: Nutritional assessment, enteral nutrition and parenteral nutrition, in Katzung BC (ed): *Clinical Pharmacology.* San Mateo, Calif, Appleton and Lang, 1988, pp 339–348.

5. Bartlett RH, et al: Measurement of metabolism in multiple organ failure. *Surgery* 1982; 92:771–779.

6. Baumgardner RN, Roche AF, Himes JH: Incremental growth tables: Supplementary to previously published charts. *Am J Clin Nutr* 1986; 43:711–722.

7. Belghiti J, et al: Impaired in vitro bacterial power of polymorphonuclear leukocyte in patients with protein calorie malnutrition. *Surg Gynecol Obstet* 1983; 154:489–492.

8. Bell SJ, Wyatt J: Nutritional guidelines for burned patients. *J Am Diet Assoc* 1986; 86:648–653.

9. Bistrian BR, et al: Cellular immunity in semi-starved states in hospitalized adults. *Am J Clin Nutr* 1975; 28:1148–1155.

10. Bistrian BR, et al: Prevalence of malnutrition in general medical patients. *JAMA* 1976; 235:1567–1570.

11. Bistrian BR, et al: Protein status of general surgical patients. *JAMA* 1974; 230:858–860.

12. Blackburn GL, et al: Indices of protein-calorie malnutrition as predictors of survival, in Sevenson SM (ed): *Nutritional Assessment—Present Status, Future Directions and Prospects.* Columbus, Ohio, Ross Laboratories, 1981, pp 131–137.

13. Blackburn GL, et al: Nutritional and metabolic assessment of the hospitalized patient. *JPEN J Parenter Enteral Nutr* 1979; 1:11.

14. Bourry V, et al: Assessment of nutritional proteins during the parenteral nutrition of cancer patients. *Ann Clin Lab Sci* 1982; 12:158–162.

15. Bozzetti F: Nutritional assessment from the perspective of a clinician. *JPEN J Parenter Enteral Nutr* 1987; 5:1155–1215.

16. Buerve KS, Mostad IL, Thoresen L: Alpha linoleic acid deficiency in patients on long-term gastric tube feeding; estimation of linoleic acid and long-chain unsaturated n-3 fatty acid requirement in man. *Am J Clin Nutr* 1987; 45:66–77.

17. Burritt MF, Anderson CR: Laboratory assessment of nutritional status. *Hum Pathol* 1984; 15:130–133.

18. Buzby GP, et al: Prognostic nutritional index in gastrointestinal surgery. *Am J Surg* 1980; 139:160–167.

19. Carpentier YA, Barthel J, Bruyns J: Plasma protein concentration in nutritional assessment. *Proc Nutr Soc* 1982; 41:405–417.

20. Chandra RK: Nutrition, immunity and infection: Present knowledge and future directions. *Lancet* 1983; 1:688–691.

21. Chandra RK: Nutritional regulation of immunity and infection in the gastrointestinal tract. *J Pediatr Gastroenterol Nutr* 1983; 1(suppl):S181–187.

22. Ching N, et al: The outcome of surgical treatment as related to the response of serum albumin level to nutritional support. *Surg Gynecol Obstet* 1980; 151:199–202.

23. Chlebowski U: Critical evaluation of the role of nutritional support with chemotherapy. *Cancer* 1985; 55:268–272.

24. Christensen KS, Gstundner KM: Hospital-wide screening improves basis for nutrition intervention. *J Am Diet Assoc* 1985; 85:704–706.

25. Clowes GHA, et al: Energy metabolism and proteolysis in traumatized and septic man. *Surg Clin North Am* 1976; 56:1169.

26. Corman LC: Effects of specific nutrients on the immune response. Selected clinical applications. *Med Clin North Am* 1985; 69:759–791.

27. Courtney ME, et al: Rapidly declining serum albumin values in newly hospitalized patients: Prevalence, severity and contributing factors. *JPEN* 1982; 6:143–145.

28. Curreri WP: Metabolic response to thermal injury and its nutritional support. *Cutis* 1978; 22:501.

29. Curreri WP: Nutritional replacement modalities. *J Trauma* 1979; 19:906.
30. Dempsey DT, et al: The link between nutritional status and clinical outcome: Can nutritional intervention modify it? *Am J Clin Nutr* 1988; 47:352–356.
31. Detsky AS, et al: Predicting nutrition-associated complications for patients undergoing gastrointestinal surgery. *JPEN* 1987; 11:440–446.
32. Detsky AS, et al: What is subjective global assessment of nutritional status? *JPEN* 1978; 11:3–13.
33. Dickerson JW: Nutrition of the cancer patient. *Adv Nutr Res* 1983; 5:105–131.
34. Dudrick SJ, et al: The effects of protein calorie malnutrition on immune competence of the surgical patient. *Surg Gynecol Obstet* 1974; 139:256–266.
35. Edwards OM, Bayless RIS, Millen S: Urinary creatinine excretions as an index of the completeness of 24-hour urine collections. *Lancet* 1969; 2:1165.
36. Elia M, Carter A, Bacon S: Clinical usefulness of urinary 3-methyl histidine excretion in indicating muscle protein breakdown. *Br Med J* [Clin Res] 1981; 282:3511–3540.
37. Elwyn DH: Nutritional requirements of adult surgical patients. *Crit Care Med* 1980; 8:9–20.
38. Faintuch J, et al: Indications and nutritional response to parenteral feeding in surgical patients with cancer. *Rev Hosp Clin Fac Med Sao Paulo* 1982; 36:194–197.
39. Feurer I, Mullen JR: Bedside measurement of resting energy expenditure and respiratory quotient via indirect calorimetry. *Nutr Clin Pract* 1986; 1:43–49.
40. Fletcher JP, et al: A comparison of serum transferrin and serum prealbumin as nutritional parameters. *JPEN* 1987; 11:144–147.
41. Forse RE, Shizgal HM: Serum albumin and nutritional status. *JPEN* 1980; 4:450.
42. Frishancho AR: New norms of upper limb fat and muscle areas for assessment of nutritional status. *Am J Clin Nutr* 1981; 34:2540–2545.
43. Garre MA, Boles JJ, Youinou PY: Current concepts in immune derangement due to undernutrition. *JPEN* 1987; 11:309–313.
44. Good RA: Nutrition and immunity. *J Clin Immunol* 1981; 1:3–11.

45. Gottschlich MM, Alexander JW: Fat kinetic and recommended dietary intake in burns. *JPEN* 1987; 11:80–85.

46. Grant J: Nutritional assessment in clinical practice. *Nutr Clin Pract* 1986; 1:3–11.

47. Grant JP, et al: Current techniques of nutritional assessment. *Surg Clin North Am* 1981; 61:437–463.

48. Gray DS, et al: Accuracy of recumbent height measurement. *JPEN* 1985; 9:712–715.

49. Griffith CDM, Ross AHM: Delayed hypersensitivity skin testing in elective colorectal surgery and relationship to postoperative sepsis. *JPEN* 1984; 8:279–280.

50. Gross RL, Newberne PM: Role of nutrition in immunologic function. *Physiol Rev* 1980; 60:188–302.

51. Hamill PVV, Drized TA, Johnson CL: Physical growth percentiles: National Center for Health Statistics. *Am J Clin Nutr* 1979; 32:607–629.

52. Heymsfield S, et al: Measurement of muscle mass in man: Validity of the 24 hour urinary creatinine method. *Am J Clin Nutr* 1989; 37:478–494.

53. Hickey MS: Enteral and parenteral nutrition, in Katzung BC (ed): *Clinical Pharmacology '89/90.* San Mateo, Calif, Appleton and Lang, in press.

54. Hickey MS, Weaver KE: Nutritional management of patients with ARC and AIDS. *Gastroenterol Clin North Am* 1988; 17:545–561.

55. Hickey MS, Weaver KE: Nutritional assessment, in Luce JM, Pierson DJ (eds): *Critical Care Medicine.* Philadelphia, WB Saunders Co, 1988, pp 355–362.

56. Hickey MS, et al: Nutrition for AIDS patients. *Contemp Surg* 1989; 35:53–79.

57. Hiebert JM, et al: The influence of catabolism of immunocompetence in burned patients. *Surgery* 1979; 86:242.

58. Hunt DR, Rowlands BJ, Johnston D: Hand grip strength: A simple prognostic indicator in surgical patients. *JPEN* 1985; 9:701–704.

59. Hunt DR, et al: A simple nutrition screening procedure for hospital patients. *J Am Diet Assoc* 1985; 85:332–335.

60. Ireton-Jones CS, Turner WW: The use of respiratory quotient to determine the efficacy of nutrition support regimens. *J Am Diet Assoc* 1987; 87:180–183.

61. Jensen TG, Englert DM, Dudrick SJ: *Nutritional Assessment: A Manual for Practitioners.* Norwalk, Conn, Appleton-Century-Crofts, 1983.

62. Jensen TG, et al: Delayed hypersensitivity skin testing: Response rates in a surgical population. *J Am Diet Assoc* 1983; 82:17–23.

63. Jensen TG, et al: Determination of nutritional status in critical care. *J Am Diet Assoc* 1984; 84:1345–1346.

64. Johnson DJ, et al: Hypothermic anesthesia attenuates postoperative proteolysis. *Ann Surg* 1986; 204:419–427.

65. Kaminski MV, et al: Correlation of mortality with serum transferrin and anergy. *JPEN* 1977; 1:27.

66. Kerpel-Frontius E: The main cause of death in malnutrition. *Acta Paediatr Hung* 1984; 25:127–130.

67. Kinney JM, et al: Indirect calorimetry in malnutrition: Nutritional assessment or therapeutic reference? *JPEN* 1987; 11(suppl):90S–94S.

68. Kirby DF, Craig RM: The value of intensive nutritional support in pancreatitis. *JPEN* 1985; 9:353–357.

69. Krey SH, Murray RL: *Dynamics of Nutrition Support.* Norwalk, Conn, Appleton-Century-Crofts, 1986.

70. Lang CE: *Nutritional Support in Critical Care.* Silver Spring, Md, American Society of Parenteral and Enteral Nutrition, 1987.

71. Law DK, Dudrick SJ, Abdou NH: The effects of protein calorie malnutrition on immune competence of the surgical patient. *Surg Gynecol Obstet* 1974; 139:257–266.

72. Law DK, et al: Immunocompetence of patients with protein-calorie malnutrition. *Ann Intern Med* 1973; 79:545–550.

73. Leff ML, et al: Resting metabolic rate: Measurement reliability. *JPEN* 1987; 11:354–359.

74. Long CL, et al: Metabolic response to injury and illness: Estimation of energy and protein needs from indirect calorimetry and nitrogen balance. *JPEN* 1979; 3:452–456.

75. Lowery SF, et al: Whole body protein breakdown and 3-methyl histidine excretion during brief fasting, starvation and intravenous repletion in man. *Ann Surg* 1985; 202:21–27.

76. Majerus TC: Nutritional support in shock and trauma. Presented at the American Society of Parenteral and Enteral Nutrition conference, San Antonio, Texas, Jan 1985.

77. Mekone TK: A new nutritional parameter. *Am Surg* 1985; 15:336–339.

78. Merkle NM, et al: Significance of the nutritional status of

surgical patients. *Lagenbecks Arch Chir* 1985; 365:109–125.

79. Messing B, Bernier JJ: Effects of two sources of energy: Nutrition ratios in patients with gastroenterological disease and malnutrition. *JPEN* 1980; 4:272–276.

80. Mirtalb JM, et al: Designing cost-effective nutritional support. *Hosp Ther* 1986; pp 56–60.

81. Mochizuki H, Trocki O, Dominioni L, et al: Mechanism of prevention of post-burn hypermetabolism and catabolism by early enteral feeding. *Ann Surg* 1984; 200:297–310.

82. Moore EE, Jones TN: Nutritional assessment and preliminary report on early support of the trauma patient. *J Am Coll Nutr* 1983; 2:45–54.

83. Moore FD: *Metabolic Care of the Surgical Patient*. Philadelphia, WB Saunders Co, 1959.

84. Mullen JL: Consequences of malnutrition in the surgical patient. *Surg Clin North Am* 1981; 61:465–485.

85. Mullen JL, et al: Implications of malnutrition in the surgical patient. *Arch Surg* 1979; 114:121–125.

86. Mullen TJ, Kirkpatrick JR: The effect of nutritional support on immune competency in patients suffering from trauma, sepsis or malignant disease. *Surgery* 1981; 90:610–615.

87. Nanni G, et al: Increased lipid fuel dependence in the critically ill septic patient. *J Trauma* 1984; 24:14–30.

88. Netland PA, Brownstein H: Anthropometric measurements for Asian and Caucasian elderly. *J Am Diet Assoc* 1985; 85:221–223.

89. Ota DM, et al: Plasma proteins as indices of response to nutritional therapy in cancer patients. *J Surg Oncol* 1985; 29:160–165.

90. Paauw JD, et al: Assessment of caloric needs of stressed patients (abstract). Proceedings of the 23rd Annual Meeting, American College of Nutrition, Arlington, Va, October 4, 1982.

91. Parker CR, Baxter CR: Divergence in adrenal steroid secretory pattern after thermal injury in adult patients. *J Trauma* 1985; 25:508–510.

92. Penzer R, Arehambeau JO: Critical evaluation of the role of nutritional support for radiation therapy patients. *Cancer* 1985; 55:263–267.

93. Peters T, Peters JC: The biosynthesis of rat serum albumin. *J Biol Chem* 1972; 247:3858.

94. Pirie P, et al: Distortion in self-reported height and weight data. *J Am Diet Assoc* 1981; 78:601–606.

95. Rennie MJ, Millward DJ: 3-Methyl histidine excretion and the urinary 3-methyl histidine/creatinine ratio are poor indication of skeletal muscle protein breakdown. *Clin Sci* 1983; 65:217–225.

96. Robinett-Weiss N, et al: The metropolitan height-weight tables: Perspectives for use. *J Am Diet Assoc* 1984; 84:1480–1481.

97. Roulet M, et al: Energy and protein metabolism in critically ill, malnourished and septic patients (abstract). *JPEN* 1980; 4:604.

98. Roy LB, et al: The value of nutritional assessment in the surgical patient. *JPEN* 1985; 9:170–172.

99. Ruberg RL: Role of nutrition in wound healing. *Surg Clin North Am* 1984; 64:705–714.

100. Saito H, et al: Metabolic and immune effects of dietary arginine supplementation after burn. *Arch Surg* 1987; 122:784–789.

101. Seltzer MH, et al: Instant nutritional assessment. *JPEN* 1979; 3:157–159.

102. Shenkin A: Assessment of nutritional status: The biochemical approach and its problems in liver disease. *J Hum Nutr* 1979; 33:341–349.

103. Shetty PS, et al: Rapid turnover transport proteins: An index of subclinical protein-energy malnutrition. *Lancet* 1979; 1:230–232.

104. Shires GT, et al: Inhibition of active sodium transport in erythrocytes from burned patients: Effect of dietary intake. *Surg Forum* 1973; 24:46.

105. Shizgal HM: Body composition and nutritional support. *Surg Clin North Am* 1981; 61:729–741.

106. Sologub VK, et al: Effect of high-calorie parenteral feeding on homeostatic indices in burned patients during the period of septicotoxemia. *Probl Gematol Pereliv Knovi* 1978; 23:5–8.

107. Solomon JR: Nutrition in the severely burned child. *Prog Pediatr Surg* 1981; 14:63.

108. Solomons NW: Functional nutritional assessment of human nutritional status: Principles and practice. *Clin Nutr* 1984; 8:151–155.

109. Soroff HS, Artz CP: An estimation of the nitrogen require-

ments for equilibrium in burned patients. *Surg Gynecol Obstet* 1961; 112:159.

110. Starker PM, et al: The response to TPN: A form of nutritional assessment. *Ann Surg* 1983; 198:720–724.

111. Starker PM, et al: Serum albumin as an index of nutritional support. *Surgery* 1982; 91:194–199.

112. Streat SJ, et al: Aggressive nutritional support does not prevent protein loss despite fat gain in septic intensive care patients. *J Trauma* 1987; 27:262–266.

113. Swinamer DL, et al: Twenty-four hour energy expenditure in critically ill patients. *Crit Care Med* 1987; 15:637–643.

114. Thompson JS, et al: Nutritional screening in surgical patients. *J Am Diet Assoc* 1984; 84:337–338.

115. Torosian MH, Daly JM: Nutritional support in the cancer-bearing host: Effects on host and tumor. *Cancer* 1986; 58:1915–1929.

116. Trocki O, et al: Effects of fish oil on post-burn metabolism and immunity. *JPEN* 1987; 11:521–528.

117. Truswell AS: Measuring nutrition. *Br Med J* 1985; 291:1258.

118. Tuten MB, et al: Utilization of prealbumin as a nutritional parameter. *JPEN* 1985; 9:709–711.

119. Van Lanschot JJ, et al: Calculation vs. measurement of total energy expenditure. *Crit Care Med* 1986; 14:981–985.

120. Weaver K, Hickey MS: Nutrition management of a malnourished patient with severe pneumocystic carinii pneumonia requiring ventilatory support. *PAACNOTES* 1989; 4:124–128.

121. Weir JR, et al: New methods for calculating metabolic rate with special reference to protein metabolism. *J Physiol* 1949; 109:1–9.

122. Weissman C, et al: Resting metabolic rate of the critically ill patient: Measured versus predicted. *J Anesthesiol* 1986; 64:673–679.

123. Wensier RL, et al: Hospital malnutrition: A prospective evaluation of general medical patients during the course of hospitalization. *Am J Clin Nutr* 1979; 32:418–426.

124. Wilmore DW: *The Metabolic Management of the Critically Ill*. New York, Plenum Medical Book Co, 1977.

125. Wilmore DW: Nutrition and metabolism following thermal injury. *Clin Plast Surg* 1974; 1:603.
126. Young GA, et al: Nutrition and delayed hypersensitivity during continuous ambulatory peritoneal dialysis in relation to peritonitis. *Nephron* 1986; 43:177–183.

KEY RECOMMENDED READINGS

For a list of key recommended readings for Chapter 1, see Appendix 2, pp. 286 and 287.

SELF-ASSESSMENT QUESTIONS

Directions. Select the best response to each of the questions or statements below and then enter the corresponding letter in the space provided.

( ) 1. What percentage of hospitalized surgical and medical patients would benefit from some form of nutritional supplementation?
   A. 10%
   B. 30%
   C. 50%
   D. 70%

   p. 1

( ) 2. A well-balanced diet for a nonstressed patient provides _____g of protein/kg/day.
   A. 0.50
   B. 0.75
   C. 1.00
   D. 2.00

   p. 1

( ) 3. One (1) g of nitrogen is equivalent to _____ g of protein.
   A. 1.50
   B. 5.50
   C. 6.25
   D. 7.00

   p. 1

( ) 4. During the hypermetabolic phase (HMP) of acute injury or illness, a patient can successfully metabolize a maximum of _____ kcal/kg.
   A. <20
   B. 30–35
   C. 35–40
   D. >40

   p. 1

( ) 5. Protein malnutrition (kwashiorkor syndrome) is characterized by all of the following, **except:**

A. Muscle atrophy
B. Impaired immunocompetence
C. Reduced serum albumin and transferrin levels
D. Consistent weight loss

p. 2

( ) 6. Protein-calorie malnutrition (marasmus syndrome) is characterized by all of the following, **except:**

A. Bradycardia
B. Hypothermia
C. Reduced basal metabolism
D. Inconsistent weight loss

p. 3

( ) 7. The body's entire glycogen reserve is consumed after _____ hours of complete starvation.

A. 10–15
B. 18–24
C. 24–36
D. 36–48

p. 4

( ) 8. The metabolism of 1 g of CHO yields approximately _____ kcal.

A. 2
B. 4
C. 6
D. 9

p. 4

( ) 9. Which energy source provides nearly 87% of the caloric requirement during a prolonged period (>24 hr) of metabolic stress and starvation?

A. Carbohydrate
B. Glycogen
C. Protein
D. Fat

p. 4

( ) 10. A nutritional assessment should include all of the following, **except:**

   A. Evaluation of protein (visceral and somatic) and fat reserve

   B. A 24-hr nitrogen balance determination

   C. Assessment of gastrointestinal function

   D. Determination of the daily caloric and protein requirements

   E. A 12-hr glucose tolerance test

   p. 5

( ) 11. Anthropometric measurements are helpful in determining the patient's _____ reserve.

   A. CHO

   B. Glycogen

   C. Fat

   D. Protein (visceral and somatic)

   p. 5

( ) 12. Nutritional therapy is usually indicated if the nutritional assessment reveals:

   A. Normal nutritional indices

   B. Normal gut function

   C. Moderate or severe malnutrition

   D. Positive nitrogen balance

   p. 6

( ) 13. A 24-hr urine collection for _____ is the most precise method for determining the degree of skeletal muscle catabolism.

   A. Arginine

   B. 3-Methyl histidine

   C. Creatinine

   D. Glutamine

   p. 2

( ) 14. The patient's gastrointestinal function should be evaluated during the initial nutritional assessment.

   A. True

   B. False

   p. 7

( ) 15. The daily caloric (kcal) requirement per kg for weight maintenance in the nonstressed, adult patient ranges from:
  A. 20–25
  B. 30–35
  C. 35–40
  D. 40–45

p. 7

( ) 16. The Harris-Benedict equation involves five variables:
  A. Height (cm), weight (kg), age (yr), activity factor and injury factor
  B. Height (cm), 24-hr nitrogen balance, age (yr), serum total protein level, and activity factor
  C. Weight (kg), 24-hr nitrogen balance, activity factor serum albumin level, and injury factor
  D. Age (yr), 24-hr nitrogen balance, activity factor, injury factor, and weight (kg)

p. 7

( ) 17. An adult male burn patient has a maintenance daily caloric requirement of 25 kcal/kg plus an additional caloric requirement of _____ kcal/% total body surface area burn/day.
  A. 20
  B. 30
  C. 40
  D. 60

p. 9

( ) 18. Malnourished ARC/AIDS patients require _____ kcal/kg/day.
  A. 25–30
  B. 30–35
  C. 35–40
  D. 45–50

p. 9

( ) 19. Malnourished AIDS/ARCS patients require _____ g of protein/kg/day.
  A. 2.0–2.5
  B. 0.8–1.0

    C. 1.0–1.5
    D. 1.5–2.0

p. 9

( ) 20. The daily caloric requirement for a nonburn, pediatric patient (age <15 yr) is dependent on _____.
    A. Age and height
    B. Age and weight
    C. Height and weight
    D. Age and sex

p. 11

( ) 21. The daily caloric requirement for nonburn pediatric patients (age >15 yr) is the same as that for nonburn adult patients.
    A. True
    B. False

p. 8

( ) 22. All of the following indicate a need for nutritional therapy, **except:**
    A. Serum albumin <2.5 g/dL
    B. Serum transferrin <150 mg/dL
    C. Total lymphocyte count <1,200/hpf
    D. Serum total protein ⩾7.5 g/dL

p. 11

( ) 23. Metabolically stressed patients should receive 75–150 nonprotein carbohydrate calories per gram nitrogen infused.
    A. True
    B. False

p. 13

( ) 24. The daily maintenance fluid (mL) requirement for a healthy, afebrile, 70-kg male ranges from:
    A. 500–1,000 cc
    B. 1,000–1,500 cc
    C. 1,500–2,000 cc
    D. 2,000–2,500 cc

p. 13

( ) 25. The maintenance fluid requirement increases
_____ % with every degree increase in temperature above normal.

A. 2%
B. 5%
C. 8%
D. 10%

p. 13

( ) 26. Patients with excessive gastric fluid losses *may* develop all of the following, **except:**

A. Hypokalemia
B. Dehydration
C. Hypochloridemia
D. Metabolic acidosis

p. 14

( ) 27. Patients with excessive small bowel fistula drainage
may develop all of the following, **except:**

A. Hypokalemia
B. Hypochloridemia
C. Dehydration
D. Metabolic alkalosis

p. 14

( ) 28. The Na, K, Cl, and HCO_3 content in mEq/L of gastric
fluid is:

A. Na = 60, K = 30, Cl = 40, HCO_3 = 0
B. Na = 60, K = 10, Cl = 130, HCO_3 = 0
C. Na = 140, K = 50, Cl = 104, HCO_3 = 30
D. Na = 100, K = 20, Cl = 100, HCO_3 = 10

p. 14

( ) 29. Enteral and parenteral diet therapy includes monitoring of the patient's blood chemistries, 24-hr nitrogen
balance, and weight.

A. True
B. False

p. 14

( ) 30. The following can result in direct, intact protein loss:
    A. Hemorrhage
    B. Pneumonia
    C. Intestinal obstruction
    D. All of the above

p. 2

( ) 31. The metabolism of 1 g of glycogen yields approximately _____ kcal.
    A. 1
    B. 2
    C. 4
    D. 9

p. 4

( ) 32. The metabolism of 1 g of protein yields approximately _____ kcal.
    A. 1
    B. 2
    C. 4
    D. 9

p. 4

( ) 33. Protein is a key component of:
    A. Enzymes
    B. Cell structure
    C. Antibodies and hormones
    D. All of the above

p. 4

( ) 34. A healthy, 70-kg individual excretes approximately _____ g of urinary nitrogen daily.
    A. 5–10
    B. 12–15
    C. 30–60
    D. 70–90

p. 4

( ) 35. Aggressive nutritional therapy, i.e., enteral or parenteral diet therapy, is not routinely required when treating patients with normal pre-illness nutritional indices who predictably can resume adequate oral food intake in 7 days.

A. True
B. False

p. 7

( ) 36. An adult, female burn patient has a maintenance daily caloric requirement of 22 kcal/kg plus an additional caloric requirement of _____ kcal/% total body surface area burn/day.

A. 10
B. 20
C. 30
D. 40

p. 7

( ) 37. The daily fluid requirement for a healthy, afebrile, 20-kg pediatric patient is approximately:

A. 1,000 cc
B. 1,500 cc
C. 2,000 cc
D. 2,500 cc

p. 13

( ) 38. The Na, K, Cl, HCO_3 content in mEq/L of pancreatic fluid is:

A. Na = 10, K = 26, Cl = 10, HCO_3 = 30
B. Na = 140, K = 5, Cl = 75, HCO_3 = 115
C. Na = 60, K = 10, Cl = 130, HCO_3 = 0
D. Na = 60, K = 30, Cl = 40, HCO_3 = 0

p. 14

( ) 39. Indirect calorimetry is more accurate than using the Harris-Benedict equation to determine the patient's daily caloric requirement.

A. True
B. False

p. 8

( ) 40. Severely malnourished patients will display minimal reactivity to antigen skin testing.

A. True
B. False

p. 11

( ) 41. A total lymphocyte count of _____ cells/hpf indicates mild malnutrition.
A. 1,200–2,000
B. 800–1,200
C. <800
D. None of the above

p. 6

( ) 42. A serum transferrin level of _____ mg/dL indicates mild malnutrition.
A. 150–200
B. 100–150
C. <100
D. None of the above

p. 6

( ) 43. The prolonged administration of a diet that delivers greater than 150 nonprotein carbohydrate calories per gram nitrogen *may* result in hepatic dysfunction.
A. True
B. False

p. 10

( ) 44. The parenteral diet of a healthy, 70-kg adult patient should provide vitamin K _____ mg weekly.
A. 1
B. 5
C. 10
D. 20

p. 12

( ) 45. The following factors may increase a patient's daily caloric requirement.
A. Infection
B. Fever
C. Surgery
D. All of the above

p. 9

( ) 46. The most sensitive indicators of the patient's response to nutritional therapy are:
  A. Serum total protein and albumin levels
  B. 24-hr nitrogen balance
  C. Weight gain
  D. Serum cholesterol level and total lymphocyte count

  p. 5

( ) 47. A precise 24-hr nitrogen balance determination should include not only urinary nitrogen losses but also losses via gastrointestinal secretions.
  A. True
  B. False

  p. 7

( ) 48. Which of the following are anthropometric measurement(s):
  A. Biceps skinfold
  B. Triceps skinfold
  C. A and B
  D. None of the above

  p. 5

( ) 49. Antigen skin testing provides a simple method for assessing the non-AIDS patient's nutritional status.
  A. True
  B. False

  p. 5

( ) 50. A patient's somatic protein reserve is evaluated by determining the:
  A. 24-hr urinary urea nitrogen excretion
  B. 24-hr urinary glutamine excretion
  C. Creatinine/height index
  D. Serum retinol building protein and pre-albumin levels

  p. 5

ENTERAL NUTRITIONAL THERAPY GUIDELINES

GENERAL DISCUSSION

Enteral diets (tube feedings) provide an inexpensive, relatively risk-free method of nutritional therapy. Most enteral diets can be administered for less than $50/day, whereas parenteral diets cost from $300 to $600/day. Enteral diets therefore are the preferred method of nutritional therapy for patients with either a functional or a semifunctional gut.

INDICATIONS FOR ENTERAL NUTRITIONAL THERAPY

Clinical Settings in Which Enteral Nutrition Should Be Part of Routine Care

Clinical settings in which enteral nutrition should be a part of routine patient care include:

- Protein-calorie malnutrition with inadequate oral nutrient intake for at least 5 days.
- Normal nutritional status (e.g., trauma patients) with less than 50% of the required nutrient intake orally for the previous 5 to 7 days.
- Severe dysphagia.
- Major full-thickness burns.
- Massive small bowel resection (in combination with the administration of total parenteral nutrition).
- Low output, low enterocutaneous fistula (mid and distal jejunum, ileal or colonic).

- Malnourished patients with acquired immune deficiency syndrome (AIDS) or AIDS-related complex (ARC).

Clinical Settings in Which Enteral Nutrition Would Usually Be Helpful

Clinical settings in which enteral nutrition would usually be helpful include:

- Major trauma.
- Radiation therapy.
- Mild chemotherapy.
- Liver and renal failure.

Clinical Settings in Which Enteral Nutrition Is of Limited or Undetermined Value

Clinical settings in which enteral nutrition is of limited or undetermined value include:

- Intensive chemotherapy.
- Immediate postoperative or post-stress period.
- Acute enteritis.
- Nonacute pancreatitis.
- Less than 10% remaining functional intestine.

CONTRAINDICATIONS TO ENTERAL NUTRITION THERAPY

Clinical settings in which nutrition therapy is contraindicated include:

- Complete mechanical intestinal obstruction.
- Ileus or intestinal hypomotility.
- Severe diarrhea.
- Low output, high enterocutaneous fistula (esophageal, gastric, duodenal, or proximal jejunum)
- High output, low or high enterocutaneous fistula.
- Acute pancreatitis.
- Shock.
- Aggressive nutritional support is not desired by the patient or legal guardian and such action is in accordance with the hospital policy and existing law.
- The patient's prognosis does not warrant aggressive nutritional support.

CLASSIFICATION OF ENTERAL DIETS

Two Major Groups of Enteral Diets

In general, enteral diets are divided into two major groups on the basis of their protein content: standard or special (Table 2–1).

Standard Diets

Standard enteral diets contain intact protein in the form of sodium and calcium caseinates, soy lactalbumin, egg albumin, or blenderized meat. They require normal gut function for maximum digestion and absorption. Consequently, standard enteral diets are indicated in the treatment of patients with normal gut function who are subjected to minimal metabolic stress. In Tables 2–2 through 2–4 a few of the more commonly administered standard enteral diets and their composition are displayed.

Special Diets

Special enteral diets (see Table 2–1) contain protein in the form of either low molecular weight free amino acids or polypeptides (Tables 2–5 and 2–6). Amino acid and polypeptide diets are readily absorbed in the presence of compromised gut function. Consequently, these diets are recommended in the treatment of patients subjected to either moderate or severe metabolic stress with compromised gut function. Also included in the special enteral diet group are the organ failure (pulmonary, renal, and hepatic) and the immuno-enriched diets. Tables 2–5 through 2–10 display a few of the more commonly administered special enteral diets and their composition.

TABLE 2–1.

Classification of Enteral Diets

Standard	Special
Intact protein, lactose-free, low-density	Free amino acid, elemental
Intact protein, lactose-free, high-density	Low molecular weight, polypeptide
Intact protein, blenderized, meat-based	Organ failure
	Pulmonary
	Renal
	Hepatic
	Immuno-enriched

TABLE 2–2.
Standard, Intact Protein, Lactose-free, Low-density (IPLFLD), Oral and Nasointestinal Enteral Diets

General Description	Nutren 1.0*	Ensure	Ensure HN	Isocal	Osmolite	Osmolite HN
kcal/mL	1.00	1.06	1.06	1.06	1.06	1.06
Protein (g/mL)	.040	.037	.044	.034	.037	.044
%kcal From fat	33.0	31.5	30.1	37.0	31.4	30.0
NPCC:N₂†	131:1	153:1	125:1	167:1	153:1	125:1
Osmolality, mOsm/kg H₂O	300	470	470	300	300	300
Trace metals: Se, Cr, Mo‡	—	—	—	NIA§	NIA§	NIA§
Glutamine (free-form)	—	—	—	—	—	—
Glutamic acid (glutamate)	+	+	+	+	+	+
BCAA content‖	NIA§	18.0	18.0	22.0	18.0 18.0	

Composition:
Carbohydrate: Maltodextrin, sucrose, corn syrup, or hydrolyzed cornstarch
Protein: Sodium and calcium caseinate, soy protein, lactalbumin, or egg albumin
Fat: Corn oil, soy oil, or medium-chain triglycerides

Clinical indications: Patients subjected to *minimal* metabolic stress with *normal* gut function (e.g., thermal [nonacute], traumatic [nonacute], or CNS [chronic] injuries; minor medical or surgical illness; and inadequate nutrient intake [chronic care or nursing home patients]).

*Recommended diet.
†NPCC:N₂ = ratio of non-protein carbohydrate to grams nitrogen.
‡Trace metals: selenium, chromium, and molybdenum.
§NIA = no information available.
‖BCAA content = branched-chain amino acid (leucine, isoleucine, and valine) content (% of the total protein content).

TABLE 2–3.

Standard, Intact Protein, Lactose-free, High-density (IPLFHD), Oral and Nasointestinal Enteral Diets

General Description	Nutren 1.5*	Nutren 2.0	Isocal HCN	Isotein HN	TwoCal HN
kcal/cc	1.50	2.00	2.00	1.20	2.00
Protein (g)/mL	.060	.080	.075	.068	.083
%kcal From fat	39.0	45.0	45.0	25.0	40.0
NPCC:N_2†	131:1	131:1	145:1	86:1	125:1
Osmolality, mOsm/kg H_2O	530	800	690	300	690
Trace metals: Se, Cr, Mo‡	—	—	—	Se, Cr, Mo	—
Glutamine (free-form)	—	—	—	—	—
Glutamic acid (glutamate)§	+	+	+	+	+
BCAA content§	NIA‖	NIA‖	23.0	22.0	21.0

Composition:

Carbohydrate: Maltodextrin, sucrose, corn syrup, or hydrolyzed cornstarch

Protein: Sodium and calcium caseinate, soy protein, lactalbumin or egg albumin

Fat: Corn oil, soy oil, or medium-chain triglycerides

Clinical indications: Patients who require fluid restriction and are subjected to *minimal* metabolic stress with *normal* gut function (e.g., thermal [nonacute], traumatic [nonacute], or CNS [acute] injuries; minor medical or surgical illness; and inadequate nutrient intake [chronic care or nursing home patients]).

*Recommended diet.

†NPCC:N_2 = ratio of non-protein carbohydrate to grams nitrogen.

‡Trace metals: selenium, chromium, and molybdenum.

§BCAA content = branched-chain amino acid (leucine, isoleucine, and valine) content (% of the total protein content).

‖NIA = no information available.

TABLE 2–4.

Standard, Intact Protein, Blenderized, Meat-based (IPBMB), Nasointestinal Enteral Diets

General Description	Compleat Modified Formula*	Compleat Regular Formula	Vitaneed
kcal/cc	1.07	1.07	1.00
Protein (g/mL)	.043	.043	.035
%kcal From fat	30.0	36.0	36.0
NPCC:N₂†	131:1	131:1	154:1
Osmolality, mOsm/kg H₂O	300	405	310
Trace metals: Se, Cr, Mo‡	Se, Cr, Mo	Se, Cr, Mo	Se, Cr, Mo
Glutamine (free-form)	—	—	—
Glutamic acid (glutamate)	+	+	+
BCAA content§	22.0	21.0	NIA‖

Composition:

Carbohydrate:	Maltodextrin, vegetables, fruit, lactose, or sucrose
Protein:	Blenderized beef, sodium and calcium caseinate, vegetables, or cereal
Fat:	Soy oil mono and triglycerides or beef fat

Clinical indications: Patients subjected to *minimal* or *moderate* metabolic stress with *normal* gut function (e.g., thermal [nonacute], traumatic [nonacute], or CNS [chronic] injuries; minor medical or surgical illness; and inadequate nutrient intake [chronic care or nursing home patients]). Also in the treatment of either (1) ARC/AIDS patients who fail elemental pure amino acid enteral diets or (2) patients who suffer from enteral diet-induced diarrhea.

*Recommended diet.
†NPCC:N₂ = ratio of non-protein carbohydrate to grams nitrogen.
‡Trace metals: selenium, chromium, and molybdenum.
§BCAA content = branched-chain amino acid (leucine, isoleucine, and valine) content (% of the total protein content).
‖NIA = no information available.

TABLE 2-5.

Special, Free Amino Acid, Elemental (FAAE), Oral and Nasointestinal Enteral Diets

General Description	Vivonex T.E.N.*	Tolerex	Stresstein
kcal/cc	1.00	1.00	1.00
Protein (g)/mL	.038	.020	.070
%kcal From fat	2.5	1.3	20.0
NPCC:N₂†	149:1	281:1	97:1
Osmolality, mOsm/kg H₂O	630	550	910
Trace metals: Se, Cr, Mo‡	Se, Cr, Mo	Se, Cr, Mo	Se, Cr, Mo
Glutamine (free-form)	+	−	+
Glutamic acid (glutamate)	−	−	−
BCAA content§	33.0	17.0	44.0

Composition:

Carbohydrate:	Maltodextrin or modified starch
Protein:	Essential and nonessential amino acids (molecular weight <500 D)
Fat:	Safflower oil, medium-chain triglycerides, or soybean oil

Clinical indications: Patients subjected to *moderate* or *severe* metabolic stress with *moderate* or *severe* gut dysfunction (e.g., thermal [acute], traumatic [acute], or CNS [acute] injuries; minor or major medical or surgical illness; immediate postoperative convalescence; low enteroenteric or enterocutaneous fistula; ARC/AIDS; malabsorption syndrome; inflammatory bowel disease; short-gut syndrome; or pancreatitis [acute or chronic]).

*Recommended diet.

†NPCC:N₂ = ratio of non-protein carbohydrate to grams nitrogen.

‡Trace metals: selenium, chromium and molybdenum.

§BCAA content = branched-chain amino acid (leucine, isoleucine, and valine) content (% of the total protein content).

TABLE 2–6.

Special, Low-molecular-weight, Polypeptide (LMWP), Nasointestinal Enteral Diets

General Description	Peptamen*	Reabilan HN	Vital HN	Pepti 2000
kcal/cc	1.00	1.33	1.00	1.00
Protein (g)/cc	.040	.057	.042	.040
%kcal From fat	33.0	35.0	9.4	8.5
NPCC:N₂†	131:1	125:1	125:1	134:1
Osmolality, mOsm/kg H₂O	260	490	500	490
Trace metals: Se, Cr, Mo‡	—	Se, Cr	NIA§	—
Glutamine (free-form)	—	—	—	—
Glutamic acid (glutamate)	+	+	+	+
BCAA content‖	23.0	NIA§	18.0	22.8
% Polypeptides MW <500 D	17	40	30–35	55

Composition:

Carbohydrate: Maltodextrin or tapioca starch

Protein: Polypeptides with variable molecular weights

Fat: Medium-chain triglycerides and long-chain triglycerides

Clinical indications: Patients subjected to *minimal* or *moderate* metabolic stress with *mild* or *moderate* gut dysfunction (e.g., minor traumatic or CNS [chronic] injuries; minor medical or surgical illness; postoperative convalescence; or pancreatitis [chronic]).

*Recommended diet.

†NPCC:N₂ = ratio of non-protein carbohydrate to grams nitrogen.

‡Trace metals: selenium, chromium, and molybdenum.

§NIA = no information available.

‖BCAA content = branched-chain amino acid (leucine, isoleucine, and valine) content (% of the total protein content).

TABLE 2–7.

Special, Pulmonary Failure (PF), Nasointestinal Enteral Diet

General Description	Pulmocare*
kcal/cc	1.50
Protein (g)/mL	.062
%kcal From fat	55.2
NPCC:N₂†	125:1
Osmolality, mOsm/kg H_2O	490
Trace metals: Se, Cr, Mo‡	NIA§
Glutamine (free-form)	—
Glutamic acid (glutamate)	+
BCAA content‖	20.7

Composition:
Carbohydrate:	Hydrolyzed cornstarch and sucrose
Protein:	Sodium and calcium caseinate
Fat:	Corn oil

Clinical indications: Patients who suffer from either acute or chronic pulmonary failure (serum CO_2 >30 mM/L) with *normal* gut function.

*Recommended diet.
†NPCC:N₂ = ratio of non-protein carbohydrate to grams nitrogen.
‡Trace metals: selenium, chromium, and molybdenum.
§NIA = no information available.
‖BCAA content = branched-chain amino acid (leucine, isoleucine, and valine) content (% of the total protein content).

Types of Enteral Diets

There are several different types of diets in both the standard and special enteral diet groups (see Table 2–1). Each type varies in

1. Carbohydrate and fat composition.
2. Caloric and protein content.
3. Ratio of non-protein carbohydrate calories to grams nitrogen.
4. Osmolality.
5. Whether or not it contains the minor trace metals selenium, chromium, and molybdenum; glutamine or glutamic acid (glutamate); or branched-chain amino acids.

TABLE 2–8.

Special, Renal Failure (RF), Nasointestinal Enteral Diets

General Description	Amin-Aid*	Travasorb Renal
kcal/cc	2.00	1.35
Protein (g)/cc	.020	.022
%kcal From fat	21.0	12.0
NPCC:N_2†	800:1	435:1
Osmolality, mOsm/kg H_2O	700	590
Trace metals: Se, Cr, Mo‡	—	—
Glutamine (free-form)	—	—
Glutamic acid (glutamate)	+	+
BCAA content§	36.0	30.6

Composition:
Carbohydrate:	Hydrolyzed cornstarch and sucrose
Protein:	Sodium and calcium caseinate
Fat:	Corn oil

Clinical indications: Patients with *normal* gut function who suffer from renal failure (serum creatinine >2.0 mg%) and who are *not undergoing routine dialysis.*

*Recommended diet.
†NPCC:N_2 = ratio of non-protein carbohydrate to grams nitrogen.
‡Trace metals: selenium, chromium, and molybdenum.
§BCAA content = branched-chain amino acid (leucine, isoleucine, and valine) content (% of the total protein content).

Important general facts regarding the content of the different types of enteral diets are discussed in the following section (**Enteral Diet Content**). The specific characteristics of the different types of standard and special enteral diets are discussed under **Types of Enteral Diets.**

ENTERAL DIET CONTENT
Carbohydrate

Enteral diets usually contain either one or a combination of the following forms of carbohydrate: maltodextrin, modified starch, sucrose, corn syrup, and/or hydrolyzed cornstarch. The specific carbohydrates present in each of the more commonly administered standard and special enteral diets are shown in Tables 2–2

TABLE 2–9.

Special, Hepatic Failure (HF), Nasointestinal Enteral Diets

General Description	Travasorb Hepatic*	Hepatic Aid II
kcal/cc	1.10	1.10
Protein (g)/cc	.025	.044
%kcal From fat	12.0	27.7
NPCC:N₂†	218:1	148:1
Osmolality, mOsm/kg H₂O	690	560
Trace metals: Se, Cr, Mo‡	—	—
Glutamine (free-form)	—	—
Glutamic acid (glutamate)	+	+
BCAA content§	50.0	46.0

Composition:
Carbohydrate:	Oligosaccharides, maltodextrin, or sucrose
Protein:	Free amino acids including branched-chain amino acids
Fat:	Medium-chain triglycerides or soybean oil

Clinical indications: Patients who suffer from hepatic failure and who *display clinical signs of encephalopathy* with *normal* gut function.

*Recommended diet.
†NPCC:N₂ = ratio of non-protein carbohydrate to grams nitrogen.
‡Trace metals: selenium, chromium, and molybdenum.
§BCAA content = branched-chain amino acid (leucine, isoleucine, and valine) content (% of the total protein content).

through 2–10. The carbohydrate content of those diets not listed in these tables are available in the *Physicians' Desk Reference.*[208]

Fat

The fat composition and content of a diet affect the patient's tolerance of the diet. Because fat provides a relatively inexpensive source of calories, enteral diets frequently contain large amounts of fat in the form of long-chain triglycerides (LCTs), medium-chain triglycerides (MCTs) or a combination of both.

Long-Chain Triglycerides

Long-chain triglycerides are poorly tolerated by patients with compromised gut function because they tend to irritate the small bowel mucosa, especially when administered in large quantities. When mucosal irritation occurs, nutrient absorption is severely limited and intraluminal fluid migration is enhanced, causing diar-

TABLE 2–10.

Special, Immuno-enriched (IE), Nasointestinal Enteral Diet

General Description	Impact*
kcal/cc	1.0
Protein (g)/cc	.06
%kcal From fat	25
NPCC:N₂†	71:1
Osmolality, mOsm/kg H₂O	375
Trace metals: Se, Cr, Mo‡	Se, Cr, Mo
Glutamine (free-form)	—
Glutamic acid (glutamate)	+
BCAA content§	17.0

Composition:

Carbohydrate:	Hydrolyzed cornstarch
Protein:	Sodium and calcium caseinates; essential and nonessential amino acids
Fat:	Palm kernel, sunflower, and menhaden oil

Clinical indications: Patients subjected to *moderate* or *severe* metabolic stress with *moderate* gut dysfunction (e.g., thermal [nonacute], traumatic [acute or nonacute], or CNS injuries; minor or major medical/surgical infections; cancer; postoperative convalescence; and HIV infection.

*Recommended diet.
†NPCC:N₂ = ratio of non-protein carbohydrate to grams nitrogen.
‡Trace metals: selenium, chromium, and molybdenum.
§BCAA content = branched-chain amino acid (leucine, isoleucine, and valine) content (% of the total protein content).

rhea. Because of the mucosal irritation, diets containing LCTs are not used in the treatment of metabolically stressed patients with compromised gut function. Instead, they are primarily used in the treatment of patients subjected to minimal metabolic stress with normal gut function.

Medium-Chain Triglycerides

In contrast, diets containing MCTs are less irritating to the small bowel mucosa and are therefore better tolerated by patients with compromised gut function. Diets containing MCTs are

1. Hydrolyzed more rapidly and completely by the intestinal lumen than those with LCT.

2. Absorbed intact by the small bowel and completely hydrolyzed by intestinal mucosal cells.
3. Transported primarily via the portal vein rather than the intestinal lymphatics.
4. Oxidized more readily than diets with LCTs.[106, 107]

The metabolic and intestinal transport of both LCTs and MCTs are shown in Figure 2–1. Because MCTs are readily absorbed and are well tolerated by patients with compromised gut function, they are recommended in the treatment of metabolically stressed patients with compromised gut function.* Table 2–11 displays the general rationale for the administration of MCTs rather than LCTs.

Total Fat Content

The total fat content of an enteral diet, in addition to the fat composition, must be considered when treating patients with gut dysfunction. Since the metabolism of 1 g of fat yields nearly 9 calories (kcal) and fats are a relatively inexpensive source of calories, many enteral diets have a relatively high fat content. In general, patients must consume 3% to 5% of their daily caloric requirement as fat to prevent the development of a fatty acid deficiency. The total calories delivered from fat therapy should not exceed 60% of the patient's estimated daily caloric requirement. Fats may be used to provide as much as 60% of the daily calories in specific clinical situations (e.g., pulmonary failure). However, if fat therapy is used to deliver more than 60% of the estimated daily caloric requirement, patients may experience compromised polymorphonuclear cells, macrophage, and reticuloendothelial cell function.*

In view of our daily fat requirement and the deleterious effect that LCTs have on the intestinal mucosa, most nutritionists prefer to administer MCT-containing diets with a total fat content of less than 5% to metabolically stressed patients with compromised gut function. The fat contents of the most commonly administered enteral diets are shown in Tables 2–2 through 2–10. Because MCTs do not contain linoleic acid, those individuals requiring extended nutritional therapy should receive supplemental free fatty acids in addition to the MCTs to prevent the development of a fatty acid deficiency. The *Physicians' Desk Reference*[208] has in-

*References 18–22, 85, 90, 106–108, 142, 171, 176, 177, 254, 258, 262.
*References 100, 163, 167, 171, 177, 178, 239.

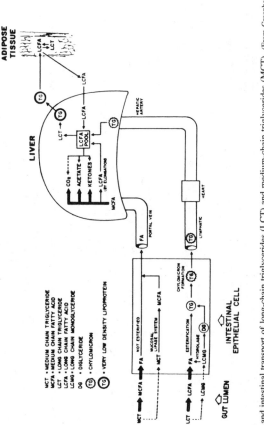

FIG 2–1.
Metabolic and intestinal transport of long-chain triglycerides (LCT) and medium-chain triglycerides (MCT). (From Greenberger NJ, Skillman TG: Medium-chain triglycerides. *N Engl J Med* 1969; 230:1045–1058. Used by permission.)

TABLE 2–11.

General Rationale for Administration of Medium-chain Triglycerides (MCTs)

Physicochemical Characteristics	Physiologic Considerations	Potential Therapeutic Applications
MCTs present more interfacial surface for enzyme action per unit time	Intraluminal enzymatic hydrolysis of MCT is more rapid and more complete than long-chain triglycerides (LCTs)	Decreased intraluminal concentrations of pancreatic lipase (pancreatic insufficiency, cystic fibrosis)
		Decreased small-bowel absorptive surface (intestinal resection)
Greater water solubility of MCT hydrolysis products	Bile salts are not required for dispersion in water	Decreased intraluminal concentrations of bile salts (intrahepatic and extrahepatic biliary tract obstruction, chronic parenchymal liver disease)
Small molecular size of MCT vs. LCT	Small amounts of MCT may enter intestinal cell without prior hydrolysis	Pancreatic insufficiency
Shorter chain length of fatty acids derived from MCT	More efficient penetration of diseased mucosal surface	Nontropical sprue, tropical sprue
Small molecular size and lower pK of fatty acids derived from MCT	Intramucosal metabolism of high-cholesterol fatty acids (HCFA) different from low-cholesterol fatty acids:	Abetalipoproteinemia
	Decreased affinity for esterifying enzymes	Hypobetalipoproteinemia
	Decreased affinity for activating enzymes	
	Minimal re-esterification of HCFA to MCT	
	No chylomicron formation	
Greater water solubility of HCFA	Different routes of transport of MCT vs. LCT:	Lymphatic obstruction (lymphomas)
	Portal transport of MCT (as HCFA)	Intestinal lymphangiectasis
	Lymphatic transport of LCT (as chylomicrons)	

From Greenberger NJ, Skillman TG: *N Engl J Med* 1969; 230:1045–1058. Used by permission.

formation regarding the fat composition and content of those enteral diets not listed in Tables 2–2 through 2–10.

Calorie and Protein

In general, most enteral diets are designed to deliver 1.0 to 1.5 kcal/cc and 0.02 to 0.04 g of protein/cc. Several of the standard, intact protein, high-density diets and a few of the special enteral diets deliver 1.5 to 2.0 kcal/mL and 0.06 to 0.08 g of protein/cc (see Tables 2–3, 2–7, and 2–10).

Ratio of Non-Protein Carbohydrate Calories to Gram Nitrogen

Enteral diets differ in their ratio of non-protein carbohydrate calories to grams nitrogen (NPCC:N_2). Because optimal caloric and protein assimilation occurs at ratios ranging from 100:1 to 150:1, most enteral diets, excluding several special organ failure diets, have NPCC:N_2 ratios within this range. Tables 2–2 through 2–10 list the NPCC:N_2 ratios of a few of the more commonly administered enteral diets, including the organ failure diets. The *Physicians' Desk Reference*[208] has information regarding the NPCC:N_2 ratios of those enteral diets not listed in these tables.

Osmolality

Enteral diets vary in their osmolality. Generally they are categorized as either isosmolar (osmolality = 280 to 300 mOsm/kg water) or hyperosmolar (osmolality >300 mOsm/kg water). The osmolality of a diet determines its infusion schedule (Table 2–12).

Isosmolar Diets

Isosmolar diets are administered routinely to patients with normal gut function who are subjected to minimal metabolic stress. Because these diets are isosmolar, they are initially infused full strength at 40 cc/hr per volumetric pump via nasointestinal feeding tube. Then, depending on the patient's estimated daily caloric and protein requirements, age, and cardiovascular status, the infusion rate is advanced according to the schedule displayed in Table 2–12.

Hyperosmolar Diets

Hyperosmolar diets are administered routinely to patients with compromised gut function who are subjected to moderate or se-

TABLE 2–12.

Enteral Diet Infusion Schedules

	Isosmolar (280–300 mOsm/kg water)	
Hours	Strength	Rate (cc/hr via pump)
12	Full	40
12	Full	80
12	Full	100–125*
	Hyperosmolar (300 mOsm/kg water)	
Hours	Strength	Rate (cc/hr via pump)
12	1/4	40
12	1/2	40
18	3/4	40
12	Full	40
12	Full	80
24	Full	100–125*

*The final infusion rate is dependent upon the patient's calculated total caloric and protein requirements, overall cardiovascular status, and tolerance of the diet.

vere metabolic stress. Because these diets are hyperosmolar, they are initially administered one-quarter strength at 40 cc/hr per volumetric pump via nasointestinal feeding tube. Then, depending on the patient's estimated daily caloric and protein requirements, age, and cardiovascular status, the infusion rate is advanced according to the schedule displayed in Table 2–12.

The osmolalities of the most commonly administered enteral diets are listed in Tables 2–2 through 2–10. The *Physicians' Desk Reference*[208] has information regarding the osmolalities of those enteral diets not mentioned in the Tables.

Major and Minor Trace Metals

Enteral diets should contain both major and minor trace metals (Table 2–13).* Most contain the major trace metals and a few of the minor trace metals. Very few diets, however, contain the important minor trace metals selenium, chromium, and molybde-

*References 8, 48, 61, 72, 81, 93, 101, 134, 148, 149, 181, 186, 210, 211, 231, 265, 266, 287, 289.

TABLE 2-13.
Trace Metals in Enteral Diets

Major Metals	Minor Metals
Calcium	Iron
Phosphorus	Copper
Magnesium	Zinc
Sodium	Iodine
Chlorine	Fluorine
Potassium	Manganese
	Selenium
	Chromium
	Molybdenum

num, which are vital for the successful recovery of metabolically stressed patients.

Selenium
Selenium has several important physiologic functions†:

1. It is an essential component of enzymes.
2. It acts as an antioxidant to help prevent cell damage.
3. It assists in the maintenance of liver integrity.

Clinically, a selenium deficiency results in muscle weakness, pain, cardiomyopathy, and possible delayed recovery from AIDS-related infections and neoplastic diseases.

Recently, Dworkin et al.[72] suggested that a selenium deficiency could affect immune and other functions vital for recovery from infectious and neoplastic diseases seen in AIDS patients. They demonstrated that there was a strong correlation between total lymphocyte count and both plasma selenium and glutathione peroxidase (G-P_x) activity (important in preventing cell damage).

Chromium
Chromium is an important trace element.[8, 48, 81, 93, 134, 148, 181] Clinically, a chromium deficiency results in

1. Impaired glucose tolerance.
2. Disturbances in protein, carbohydrate, and lipid metabolism.

†References 8, 72, 101, 148, 149, 265, 266, 289.

3. Neuropathy.
4. Weight loss.

Chromium is also a key component of the glucose tolerance factor (GTF). During the hypermetabolic phase (HMP) of acute illness or injury, glucose metabolism (serum clearance) is normally reduced, resulting in elevated serum glucose levels. A reduction in GTF secondary to a chromium deficiency further reduces glucose metabolism during the HMP.

Molybdenum

Molybdenum, like selenium, is an essential component of several enzyme systems.[8, 48, 63, 148, 181, 277] Clinically, a molybdenum deficiency results in

1. Amino acid intolerance.
2. Irritability.
3. Lethargy.
4. Coma.
5. Headache.

Tables 2–2 through 2–10 indicate which of the most commonly administered enteral diets contain the important minor trace metals selenium, chromium, and molybdenum. The *Physicians' Desk Reference*[208] has information regarding the trace metal content of those enteral diets not mentioned in the Tables.

Glutamine

Enteral diets should contain glutamine supplements, especially those used in the treatment of patients subjected to either moderate or severe metabolic stress. Glutamine is a nonessential neutral amino acid that can be synthesized by virtually all tissues in the body. It has several unique properties which suggest that it plays an important role in the metabolically stressed patient:

1. Glutamine is the most abundant amino acid in whole blood with concentrations in the basal state of approximately 600 to 650 mol/L.[13, 33, 79, 80, 241, 282]

2. Of those amino acids incorporated into protein, glutamine is the most abundant one in the intracellular free amino acid pool.[33, 197] Excluding taurine, glutamine constitutes 61% of the amino acid pool in skeletal muscle and exists in humans at a concentration of 20 mmol/L in intracellular water,[23] which is 30

times greater than the whole blood concentration. Given that this pool and skeletal muscle constitute 70% to 80% of the entire body's free amino acid pool,[198] it can be calculated that glutamine comprises half of the whole body pool of all free amino acids.

3. Glutamine and alanine transport more than half of the circulating amino acid nitrogen.[223, 242] These two amino acids comprise more than 50% of the amino acids released from skeletal muscle and the postabsorptive state[79, 80, 228] and possibly following injury.[139] Because glutamine has two nitrogen moieties, it is the principal carrier of nitrogen from the periphery to the visceral organs.

4. Glutamine concentrations in whole blood and skeletal muscle decrease markedly following injury and other catabolic diseases.[139, 197, 241, 246, 255] Following injury,[14, 15] operation,[139, 271] and sepsis,[222, 223] more than half of intracellular glutamine stores may be depleted, while plasma levels fall 20 to 30%. The decline in glutamine concentrations exceeds that of any other amino acid and persists during recovery after all other amino acid concentrations have returned to normal.[14, 15] In addition, the intraorgan flux of glutamine is significantly altered in disease states.[241, 244, 245]

Glutamine is avidly consumed by replicating cells such as fibroblasts,[291] lymphocytes,[2] tumor cells,[216] and intestinal epithelial cells.[281-283, 285] These cells have high glutaminase activity and low levels of intracellular glutamine. This may be of significance in patients with large wounds, inflammation associated with infection, or gastrointestinal dysfunction which precludes enteral feeding.[248]

Catabolic disease states such as trauma, sepsis, major burns, and uncontrolled diabetes are characterized by accelerated skeletal muscle proteolysis and translocation of amino acids from the periphery to the visceral organs.[150, 197, 241, 244, 245, 279] Glutamine accounts for a major portion of the amino acids released by muscle during stress states.[139, 197, 241] Despite accelerated skeletal muscle release during critical illness, the circulating concentration of glutamine is diminished,[139, 197, 241, 244, 245] indicating that accelerated uptake occurs in other tissues. A number of recent studies have demonstrated that glutamine consumption by the intestinal tract in vivo is markedly increased following operation,[241, 244] bacteremia, or glucocorticoid treatment.[241, 242, 245]

Glutamine uptake in the gastrointestinal tract occurs in the epithelial cells that line the villi of the small bowel.[199, 282, 283, 285]

Glutamine metabolism by the small intestine (1) provides a major energy source for the gut *and* (2) processes nitrogen and carbon from other tissue into the precursors for hepatic ureagenesis and gluconeogenesis.

In addition to being the preferential energy substrate for the small bowel mucosa, glutamine may also play an important role in maintaining normal intestinal structure and function.[204]

Because glutamine is the preferential energy substrate of the small bowel mucosa and it apparently has a significant role in maintaining intestinal structure and function, enteral diets fortified with glutamine are recommended when treating metabolically stressed patients with normal or compromised gut function. Because glutamine is directly absorbed into and utilized by the cell mitochondria, in contrast to glutamic acid (glutamate), glutamine rather than glutamic acid (glutamate) fortified enteral diets are recommended.[155]

Branched-Chain Amino Acids

Enteral diets may contain branched-chain amino acids (BCAA) (leucine, isoleucine, and valine). The value of BCAA-fortified enteral diets remains controversial. Brennan et al.[41] discovered in their clinical studies that while positive results in the parameters of nitrogen metabolism have been observed when administering BCAA-enriched solutions to critically ill patients, little major effect on overall outcome has yet to be demonstrated.

In contrast, Cerra et al.[51, 52] have been able to favorably modulate metabolic response to stress with an alternative fuel, i.e., BCAA-fortified diets. Their studies have clearly demonstrated the beneficial effect of BCAA on nitrogen balance under stress conditions through effects on both protein synthesis and degradation. Their findings are consistent with the observations of several other investigators.*

Because BCAA are rapidly consumed during periods of metabolic stress and there are substantial data supporting their beneficial effect on protein synthesis and degradation, BCAA-fortified diets are recommended in the treatment of patients subjected to either moderate or severe metabolic stress. The optimal dietary concentration of BCAA, however, has not been determined.

*References 28, 56, 91, 92, 125, 165, 203, 235.

TYPES OF ENTERAL DIETS

There are seven types of enteral diets:

1. Standard, intact protein, lactose-free, low-density, oral and nasointestinal.
2. Standard, intact protein, lactose-free, high-density, oral and nasointestinal.
3. Standard, intact protein, blenderized, meat-based, nasointestinal.
4. Special, free amino acid, elemental, oral and nasointestinal.
5. Special, low molecular weight, polypeptide, nasointestinal.
6. Special, organ failure: pulmonary, renal, and hepatic nasointestinal.
7. Immuno-enriched, nasointestinal.

Table 2–14 lists the seven types, identifies the most commonly administered brands in each type, and displays their basic composition. The composition and clinical indications for each type of diet are briefly discussed in the following section and summarized in Tables 2–2 through 2–10.

Standard, Intact Protein, Lactose-Free, Low-Density (IPLFLD), Oral and Nasointestinal Enteral Diets

These diets (e.g., Nutren 1.0, Ensure, Ensure HN, Isocal, Osmolite, and Osmolite HN) are standard diets that require normal gut function for maximum absorption and utilization (see Table 2–1).[208] They contain

- Protein in the form of sodium and calcium caseinates, soy, lactalbumin, or egg albumin.
- Carbohydrate as maltodextrin, sucrose, corn syrup, or hydrolyzed cornstarch.
- Fat as corn oil, soy oil, or MCT.

IPLFLD diets

- Provide 1.0 to 1.5 kcal/cc.
- Are lactose-free.
- Have NPCC:N_2 ratios that range from 125 to 167:1.

TABLE 2–14.
Enteral Diet Characteristics

Name	kcal/cc	NPCC:N_2 Ratio*	mOsm/kg H_2O	gm Protein/cc	gm fat/cc	Na, mEq/cc	K, mEq/cc
Intact protein/lactose-free							
Nutren 1.0†	1.00	131:1	300	.040	.038	.022	.032
Ensure	1.06	153:1	450	.037	.037	.037	.040
Ensure HN	1.06	125:1	470	.044	.035	.040	.040
Isocal	1.06	167:1	300	.034	.044	.023	.034
Osmolite	1.06	153:1	300	.037	.038	.028	.026
Osmolite HN	1.06	125:1	310	.044	.037	.040	.040
Intact protein/lactose-free/high density							
Nutren 1.5†	1.50	131:1	410	.060	.068	.033	.048
Nutren 2.0†	2.00	131:1	710	.080	.106	.044	.064
Isocal HCN	2.00	145:1	690	.075	.091	.035	.036
Isotein HN	1.20	86:1	300	.068	.034	.027	.027
TwoCal HN	2.00	126:1	740	.083	.091	.046	.059
Blenderized meat-based							
Compleat Modified Formula†	1.07	131:1	300	.043	.037	.029	.036
Compleat Regular Formula	1.07	131:1	405	.043	.043	.056	.036
Vitaneed	1.00	154:1	310	.035	.040	.022	.032

Free amino acid							
Vivonex T.E.N.†	1.00	149:1	630	.038	.003	.020	.020
Tolerex	1.00	281:1	550	.020	.001	.020	.030
Stresstein	1.20	97:1	910	.070	.028	.028	.028
Polypeptide							
Peptamen†	1.00	131:1	270	.040	.039	.022	.032
Reabilan HN	1.33	125:1	490	.058	.052	.043	.042
Vital HN	1.00	125:1	460	.041	.011	.020	.034
Pepti 2000	1.00	156:1	490	.040	.010	.029	.029
Specific organ failure							
Pulmonary							
NutriVent	1.50	115:2	450	.068	.095	.033	.057
Pulmocare†	1.50	125:1	490	.062	.092	.057	.049
Renal							
Travasorb Renal†	1.35	363:1	590	.023	.018	—	—
Amin-Aid	2.00	830:1	1095	.019	.046	<.015	<.006
Hepatic							
Travasorb Hepatic†	1.10	218:1	600	.029	.015	.010	.023
Hepatic-Aid	1.10	148:1	560	.044	.036	<.015	<.006
Immuno-enriched							
Impact†	1.0	71:1	375	.060	.028	.047	.033

*Ratio of non-protein calories to grams nitrogen.
†Recommended

- Have osmolalities that range from 300 to 470 mOsm/kg water.

They are often deficient in selenium, chromium, molybdenum, glutamine, and glutamic acid (glutamate). IPLFLD diets derive between 30% and 70% of their calories from fat metabolism, and 20% of the total protein content may be in the form of BCAA. Because of their composition, IPLFLD diets are recommended only in the treatment of patients subjected to minimal metabolic stress and with normal gut function, for example:

- Thermal (nonacute), traumatic (nonacute), or central nervous system CNS (chronic) injuries.
- Minor medical or surgical illness.
- Inadequate nutrient intake (chronic care or nursing home patients).

Several of these diets may be administered both orally and via nasointestinal feeding tube. Tables 2–2 and 2–14 summarize the important characteristics of the IPLFLD diets.

Standard, Intact Protein, Lactose-Free, High-Density (IPLFHD), Nasointestinal Enteral Diets

These enteral diets (e.g., Nutren 1.5, Nutren 2.0, Isocal HCN, Isotein HN, and TwoCal HN) are standard diets that also require normal gut function for maximum absorption and utilization (see Table 2–1).[208] They contain essentially the same protein, carbohydrate, and fat as IPLFLD diets. They differ from IPLFLD diets in that they are more concentrated. IPLFHD diets

- Provide 1.2 to 2.0 kcal/cc.
- Are lactose-free.
- Have NPCC:N_2 ratios that range from 86 to 145:1.
- Have osmolalities that range from 300 to 740 mOsm/kg of water.

They are often deficient in selenium, chromium, molybdenum, glutamine, and glutamic acid (glutamate). IPLFHD diets derive between 25% and 40% of their calories from fat metabolism, and 20% to 22% of the total protein content may be in the form of BCAA. They are recommended in the treatment of patients subjected to minimal metabolic stress with normal gut function who require fluid restriction, e.g.,

- Thermal (nonacute), traumatic (nonacute), or CNS (acute) injuries.
- Minor medical or surgical illness.
- Inadequate nutrient intake (chronic care or nursing home patients).

These diets are routinely administered via nasointestinal feeding tube. The important characteristics of the IPLFHD diets are summarized in Tables 2–3 and 2–14.

Standard, Intact Protein, Blenderized, Meat-Based (IPBMB), Nasointestinal Enteral Diets

These enteral diets (e.g., Compleat Modified Formula, Compleat Regular Formula, and Vitaneed) are standard diets that require normal gut function for maximum absorption and utilization (see Table 2–1).[208] IPBMB diets contain

- Protein in the form of blenderized beef.
- Carbohydrate as maltodextrin, vegetables, fruit, lactose, or sucrose.
- Fat as soy oil, mono and triglycerides, or beef fat.

IPBMB diets

- Provide 1.0 to 1.07 kcal/cc.
- Have NPCC:N_2 ratios that range from 131 to 154:1.
- Have osmolalities that range from 300 to 405 mOsm/kg water.
- Contain pectin

Compleat Modified Formula and Compleat Regular Formula contain selenium, chromium, and molybdenum. These diets also contain either glutamine or glutamic acid (glutamate). IPBMB diets derive between 30% and 36% of their calories from fat metabolism, and 20% to 22% of the total protein content is in the form of BCAA. They are recommended in the treatment of patients subjected to minimal or moderate metabolic stress with normal gut function, e.g.,

- Thermal (nonacute), traumatic (nonacute), or CNS (chronic) injuries.
- Minor medical or surgical illness.
- Inadequate nutrient intake (chronic care or nursing home patients).

IPBMB diets are also used in the treatment of (1) patients with acquired immune deficiency syndrome (AIDS) or AIDS-related complex (ARC) who fail a free amino acid, elemental or polypeptide enteral diet *and* (2) patients who suffer from enteral diet–induced diarrhea. These diets are routinely administered by means of a nasointestinal feeding tube. The important characteristics of IPBMB diets are summarized in Tables 2–4 and 2–14.

Special, Free Amino Acid, Elemental (FAAE), Oral and Nasointestinal Enteral Diets

These enteral diets (e.g., Vivonex T.E.N., Tolerex, and Stresstein) are special diets that are readily absorbed in the presence of either moderate or severe gut dysfunction (see Table 2–1).[208] The FAAE diets contain

- Protein in the form of low molecular weight (MW) free amino acids (MW <500 D).
- Carbohydrate as maltodextrin and modified starch.
- Fat as safflower oil, soybean oil, or MCT.

FAAE diets

- Provide 1.0 to 1.2 kcal/cc.
- Have NPCC:N_2 ratios that range from 97 to 281:1.
- Have osmolalities that range from 550 to 910 mOsm/kg of water.

They contain adequate amounts of selenium, chromium, and molybdenum as well as all of the other major and minor trace metals. Vivonex T.E.N. and Tolerex contain glutamine. Stresstein contains glutamic acid (glutamate). The FAAE diets derive less than 3% of their calories from fat metabolism, and 16% to 44% of the total protein content is in the form of BCAA. Because of their protein, trace metal, glutamine, fat, and BCAA content, FAAE diets are highly recommended in the treatment of patients subjected to moderate or severe metabolic stress with either normal or compromised gut dysfunction,* e.g.,

- Thermal (acute), traumatic (acute), or CNS (acute) injuries.
- Minor or major medical or surgical illness.
- Immediate postoperative convalescence.
- Low enteroenteric or enterocutaneous fistula.

*References 11, 12, 117, 121, 147, 191, 207, 213, 214, 260, 261.

- ARC and AIDS malabsorption syndrome.
- Inflammatory bowel disease.
- Short gut syndrome.
- Pancreatitis (acute or chronic).

Many of these diets may be administered both orally and via nasointestinal feeding tube. Tables 2–5 and 2–14 summarize the important characteristics of FAAE diets.

Special, Low Molecular Weight, Polypeptide (LMWP), Nasointestinal Enteral Diets

These enteral diets (e.g., Peptamen, Reabilan HN, Vital HN, and Pepti 2000) are special diets which are readily absorbed in the presence of either mild or moderate gut dysfunction (see Table 2–1).[208] LMWP diets contain

- Protein in the form of polypeptides (variable molecular weights).
- Carbohydrate as maltodextrin or tapioca starch.
- Fat as LCT or MCT.

These diets

- Provide 1 kcal/cc.
- Have NPCC:N_2 ratios that range from 125 to 175:1.
- Have osmolalities that range from 260 to 490 mOsm/kg of water.

LMWP diets often lack selenium, chromium, molybdenum, glutamine, and glutamic acid (glutamate). LMWP diets derive between 8.5 to 35% of their calories from fat metabolism and contain 18% to 23% BCAA. They are recommended in the treatment of patients subjected to minimal or moderate metabolic stress [145, 146] with mild or moderate gut dysfunction, e.g.,

- Minor traumatic or CNS (chronic) injuries.
- Minor medical or surgical illness.
- Postoperative convalescence.
- ARC/AIDS.
- Pancreatitis (chronic).

These diets are routinely administered via a nasointestinal feeding tube. The important characteristics of LMWP diets are summarized in Tables 2–6 and 2–14.

Special, Pulmonary Failure (PF), Nasointestinal Enteral Diet

Pulmocare is a special (see Table 2–1) pulmonary failure (PF), nasointestinal enteral diet.[208] It has a relatively high fat content (55% of the total calories) in comparison with other enteral diets. Because the respiratory quotient (R/Q) for fat metabolism is 0.7 and the R/Q for carbohydrate metabolism is 1.0, Pulmocare should, in theory, lower the serum CO_2.

Pulmocare

- Provides 1.5 kcal/cc.
- Has an NPCC:N_2 ratio of 125:1.
- Has an osmolality of 490 mOsm/kg water.

Information regarding the selenium, chromium and molybdenum content of Pulmocare is not currently available. It contains glutamic acid (glutamate) rather than glutamine. Because Pulmocare has a high fat content (corn oil) and contains standard protein (sodium and calcium caseinates), it is recommended in the treatment of patients with either acute or chronic pulmonary failure (serum CO_2 >30 mEq/L) and normal gut function.[16, 26, 130, 151, 199, 280] These diets are routinely administered by way of a nasointestinal feeding tube. The important characteristics of PF diets for adults are summarized in Tables 2–7 and 2–14.

Special, Renal Failure (RF), Nasointestinal Enteral Diets

Travasorb Renal and Amin-Aid are special (see Table 2–1) renal failure (RF) nasointestinal enteral diets.[208] Renal failure diets contain

- Only essential amino acids or a combination of both essential and nonessential amino acids.
- A high concentration of carbohydrate as glucose oligosaccharides, sucrose, maltodextrin, or sucrose.
- Fat as MCT, sunflower oil, or partially hydrogenated soybean oil.
- Negligible concentrations of sodium, potassium, phosphorus, and calcium.

Renal failure diets

- Provide 1.35 to 2.0 kcal/cc.
- Have NPCC:N_2 ratios that range from 262 to 830:1.

- Have osmolalities that range from 590 to 1,095 mOsm/kg of water.

There is no information available regarding the selenium, chromium, and molybdenum contents of these diets. Renal failure diets contain glutamic acid (glutamate). They derive between 12% and 21% of their calories from fat metabolism, and 29% to 39% of the protein content is in the form of BCAA. They are indicated in the treatment of patients with normal gut function who suffer from renal failure (serum creatinine >2.0 mg%) and who are *not undergoing routine dialysis*. They are contraindicated in the treatment of patients with compromised gut function or *undergoing routine dialysis*. These diets are routinely administered via nasointestinal feeding tube. The important characteristics of RF diets are summarized in Tables 2–8 and 2–14.

Special, Hepatic Failure (HF), Nasointestinal Enteral Diets

Travasorb Hepatic and Hepatic-Aid II are special (see Table 2–1) hepatic failure nasointestinal diets.[208] Hepatic failure diets contain

- Primarily BCAA.
- A high concentration of carbohydrate as glucose oligosaccharide, maltodextrin, or sucrose.
- Fat as partially hydrogenated soybean oil, sunflower oil, or MCT.
- Negligible concentrations of sodium, potassium, phosphorus, and calcium.

These diets

- Provide 1.1 kcal/cc.
- Have NPCC:N_2 ratios that range from 148 to 218:1.
- Have osmolalities that range from 560 to 690 mOsm/kg water.

There is no information regarding their selenium, chromium, and molybdenum contents; they contain glutamic acid (glutamate), derive 12% to 28% of their calories from fat metabolism, and 46% to 50% of their protein content is in the form of BCAA. They are indicated in the treatment of patients with normal gut function who suffer from hepatic failure and who *display clinical signs of encephalopathy*. They are contraindicated in the treatment of patients with compromised gut function or *without encephalopathy*. These diets are routinely administered by means of a nasointestinal feeding tube. The characteristics of HF diets are summarized in Tables 2–9 and 2–14.

Special, Immuno-Enriched (IE), Nasointestinal Enteral Diet

Impact is a special (see Table 2–1), immuno-enriched (IE), nasointestinal enteral diet.[208] Impact has been specially formulated to stimulate the immune system and provide an excellent source of nutrition for patients subjected to moderate or severe metabolic stress with mild to moderate gut dysfunction. It contains

- Arginine, which strongly stimulates lymphocyte reactivity in healthy humans.[24, 64, 225, 226, 273]
- Additional ribonucleic acid, which is vital for monitoring normal cellular immunity and host resistance.[77, 157, 263, 264]
- Additional omega-3 fatty acids and decreased omega-6 fatty acids, which are beneficial in improving the survival of patients at risk for infection.
- Structured lipids composed of MCTs and LCTs, which provide essential fatty acids in a form that is rapidly transported and utilized.[24, 64]

Impact

- Contains protein in the form of essential and nonessential amino acids and sodium and calcium caseinates.
- Carbohydrate as hydrolyzed cornstarch.
- Fat as palm kernel, sunflower, and refined menhaden oil.

It

- Provides 1.0 kcal/cc.
- Has an NPCC:N_2 ratio of 71:1.
- Has an osmolality of 375 mOsm/kg of water.

Impact contains selenium, chromium, molybdenum, and glutamic acid (glutamate). It derives approximately 25% of its calories from fat metabolism, and 17% of its protein content is in the form of BCAA.

Impact is highly recommended in the treatment of patients subjected to moderate or severe metabolic stress with normal or compromised gut function, e.g.,

- Thermal (nonacute), traumatic (acute or nonacute) or CNS injuries.
- Minor or major medical/surgical infection.
- Cancer.
- Postoperative convalescence.
- Human immunodeficiency virus (HIV) infection.

Impact is routinely administered by means of a nasointestinal feeding tube. The characteristics of Impact are summarized in Tables 2–10 and 2–14.

ENTERAL DIET ADMINISTRATION
General Facts

Enteral diets are routinely infused through a nasointestinal feeding tube. The position of the tube in the small bowel lumen must be confirmed by abdominal x-ray prior to starting the infusion of the diet. Enteral diets are infused continuously by means of a volumetric pump. Bolus and gravity feedings are not recommended because of the risk of aspiration. Table 2–15 is a list of the various types of enteral feeding tubes; Table 2–16 shows the

TABLE 2–15.

Types of Enteral Feeding Tubes

Nasogastric	Nasointestinal	Percutaneous Gastrostomy	Jejunostomy
No. 8 or no. 5 Infant Feeding Tube*	EnTube*	Wills-Oglesby*	No. 8 or no. 5 Infant Feeding Tube*
No. 8 Salem Sump	Ring-McLean*	Glaser Peg	Biosearch Needle Jejunostomy
	Dobhoff		Biosearch K-Tube
	Flexiflo		
	Ethox		
	Endo-Tube		
	Moss		
	Pedi-Tube		

*Recommended.

TABLE 2-16.

Administration of Enteral Diets

Route	Method	Pump
Nasogastric*	Continuous infusion per volumetric pump*	Compat*
Nasointestinal*		Kangaroo 224
Percutaneous gastrostomy*		
Jejunostomy*		

*Recommended.

routes, methods, and pumps used to administer enteral diets. The non-protein carbohydrate calories and protein delivered by the various enteral diets over 24 hours when administered at specific concentrations and hourly infusion rates are displayed in Table 2-17.

Isosmolar Diets

The infusion schedule for an enteral diet is dependent on its osmolality. Isosmolar diets are initially infused full strength at a rate of 40 cc/hr per volumetric pump. Then, as tolerated, the infusion rate is advanced according to the schedule displayed in Table 2-12. The final infusion rate is dependent on the patient's estimated daily caloric and protein requirements, age, and cardiovascular status (see Chapter 1).

Hyperosmolar Diets

Hyperosmolar diets, in contrast to isosmolar diets, are initially infused one-quarter strength at a rate of 40 cc/hr per volumetric pump. Then, as tolerated, the infusion rate is advanced according to the schedule displayed in Table 2-12. The final infusion rate is dependent on the patient's estimated daily caloric and protein requirements, age, and cardiovascular status (see Chapter 1).

Standard Enteral Nutrition Therapy Orders

Standard enteral nutrition therapy orders are simple to write and should indicate not only the diet selection but also give explicit therapeutic monitoring guidelines. Routine enteral therapy orders should include the following:

1. Insert a nasointestinal feeding tube.
2. Request a STAT portable KUB following insertion of the tube to confirm its position in the small bowel. Notify the physician when the KUB is completed.
3. Begin _____ (enteral diet) at (strength) at _____ cc/hr continuously by volumetric pump via the nasointestinal feeding tube when notified by the physician that the feeding tube is positioned in the small bowel.
4. Elevate the head of the bed 30 degrees or more while administering the enteral diet.
5. Administer only liquid medications or powdered solids suspended in liquid by a pharmacist are administered via the feeding tube.
6. Flush the feeding tube every 4 hr with 20 cc of sterile water.
7. Check for residuals every 4 hr. If the residual is >150 cc, discontinue the infusion for 2 hr. After 2 hr, recheck for residual. If the residual is <150 cc, restart the enteral diet infusion. If the residual remains >150 cc, do not restart the infusion until the physician is notified.
8. Notify the physician for persistent residuals >150 cc, increasing abdominal distention, nausea, vomiting, diarrhea, or an oral temperature >38° C.
9. Maintain strict input/output records (I/O) every shift. Total the I/O every 24 hr.
10. Record the patient's weight weekly in kilograms on the vital signs sheet.
11. Check the urine for sugar and acetone every shift and record on the vital signs sheet. If the urine sugar is 4+, request a STAT serum glucose test. If the serum glucose level is >160 mg%, contact the physician for treatment orders.
12. Administer (via nasointestinal feeding tube):
    Neutra-Phos (phosphate supplement): 1 to 2 caps (250 mg/cap) dissolved in 75 to 150 cc of the enteral diet four times daily
    Zinc sulfate (zinc supplement): 200 mg added to the enteral diet twice daily
    Titralac (calcium supplement): 2 tsp added to the enteral diet twice daily

TABLE 2–17.

Non-protein Calories (NPC)* and Protein (P) Delivered by the Various Enteral Diets When Administered at a Specific Concentration and Infusion Rate†

Enteral Diet Strength	1/4			1/2			3/4			Full		
(infusion rate, cc/hr)	(40)	(80)	(125)	(40)	(80)	(125)	(40)	(80)	(125)	(40)	(80)	(125)
Vivonex T.E.N.												
NPC:	204	408	632	404	808	1,252	608	1,216	1,884	812	1,624	2,516
P:	9	18	28	19	38	59	28	56	87	37	74	115
Peptamen												
NPC:	200	404	630	404	808	1,260	604	1,208	1,890	808	1,612	2,520
P:	10	19	30	19	38	60	29	58	90	38	77	120
Compleat Modified Formula												
NPC:	217	434	673	430	860	1,333	646	1,292	2,003	863	1,726	2,676
P:	10	20	31	21	42	65	31	62	96	41	82	127
Ensure HN												
NPC:	211	422	655	421	842	1,306	636	1,276	1,972	842	1,692	2,624
P:	11	22	34	22	44	68	36	64	99	43	86	133
Nutren 1.0												
NPC:	200	404	630	404	808	1,260	604	1,208	1,890	808	1,612	2,520
P:	10	19	30	19	38	60	29	58	90	38	77	120
Isocal												
NPC:	253	446	691	441	882	1,368	664	1,328	2,056	886	1,972	2,718
P:	8	16	25	17	34	53	25	50	78	33	66	102

Product												
Osmolite NPC:	219	438	679	437	874	1,354	656	1,312	2,036	874	1,748	2,708
P:	9	18	28	18	36	56	27	54	84	36	72	112
Nutren 1.5 NPC:	304	606	945	605	1,208	2,250	908	1,816	2,520	1,208	2,420	3,780
P:	14	29	45	29	58	90	43	86	135	58	115	180
Nutren 2.0 NPC:	404	808	1,260	808	1,616	2,520	1,208	2,416	3,780	1,616	3,224	5,040
P:	19	38	60	38	76	120	58	116	180	76	154	240
Isocal HCN NPC:	408	816	1,264	816	1,632	2,528	1,224	2,448	3,796	1,632	3,324	5,060
P:	18	36	56	36	72	112	54	108	167	72	144	223
Pulmocare NPC:	300	600	928	600	1,200	1,860	900	1,800	2,788	1,200	2,400	3,720
P:	15	30	47	30	60	93	45	90	140	60	120	186
Travasorb Renal NPC:	300	604	945	624	1,252	1,885	904	1,812	2,830	1,208	2,416	3,774
P:	6	11	17	12	23	35	17	33	52	22	44	69
Travasorb Hepatic NPC:	236	472	737	472	944	1,474	708	1,416	2,215	944	1,888	2,952
P:	7	14	22	14	28	49	21	42	65	28	56	87
Impact NPC:	240	480	744	480	960	1,488	720	1,440	2,232	960	1,920	2,976
P:	14	28	43	29	58	90	43	86	133	58	116	180

*1 g of glucose yields 3.34 calories.

†The NPCC and P values above are based on the indicated concentration and hourly infusion rate administered over 24 hours.

13. Routine enteral diet laboratory specimens are to be drawn weekly on the day and the time specified below:
    Thursday A.M.: Complete blood count, SMAC-20, copper, zinc, magnesium, transferrin, triglyceride, prealbumin, and retinol binding protein
14. All changes in the enteral diet therapy must be approved by the physician.

ANTIDIARRHEAL THERAPY
General Facts

Patients receiving oral or nasointestinal enteral diet therapy often develop diarrhea. The diarrhea is usually caused by one or a combination of the following:

1. Polypharmacy (e.g., multiple antibiotics).
2. Mechanical gut dysfunction (e.g., partial small bowel obstruction).
3. Intestinal bacterial overgrowth (e.g., *Clostridium difficile*).
4. Enteral diets:
   a. Composition:
      (1) Protein: intact protein vs. amino acid vs. polypeptide.
      (2) Carbohydrate.
      (3) Fat: MCTs vs. LCTs.
   b. Content:
      (1) Protein.
      (2) Carbohydrate.
      (3) Fat.
   c. Concentration.
   d. Infusion rate.
5. Intrinsic bowel disease (e.g., inflammatory bowel disease).
6. Systemic disease (e.g., HIV infection, amyloidosis, or systemic lupus erythematosus).
7. Hypoalbuminemia (serum albumin <2.5 g/dL).

Treatment Algorithm

Oral or enteral diet-induced diarrhea is usually the result of

- Polypharmacy.
- Mechanical gut dysfunction.
- Intestinal bacterial overgrowth.
- The enteral diet's composition, content, concentration, or infusion rate.

Frequently, this condition can be successfully treated by

- Eliminating specific medications.
- Correcting the gut dysfunction.
- Administering appropriate antibiotics.
- Changing the enteral diet.
- Altering the diet's administration (i.e., infusion rate).

In addition, antidiarrheal agents, administered either enterally or parenterally (see the section **Antidiarrheal Agents**), are very helpful in controlling the diarrhea.

Patients with diarrhea secondary to intrinsic bowel disease, systemic disease, or hypoalbuminemia are more difficult to treat. They require disease specific chemotherapy and possibly albumin replacement therapy (see the section **Albumin Replacement Therapy**) in addition to antidiarrheal agents.

Antidiarrheal Agents

Of the several antidiarrheal agents available, the most commonly administered include Lomotil, Imodium, deodorized tincture of opium (DTO), and Sandostatin.

Lomotil

Lomotil (manufactured by G.D. Searle & Co., Chicago, Ill)[208] is classified as a Schedule V controlled substance by federal law. It has an anticholinergic effect upon gut peristalsis. It is an excellent antidiarrheal agent for non-AIDS patients with mild to moderate diarrhea. Lomotil is administered as follows:

Oral	1 to 2 tablets (2.5 mg/tab) orally every 6 hr prn
Nasointestinal feeding tube	5 to 10 cc (2.5 mg/cc) every 4–6 hr prn

Imodium

Imodium (manufactured by Janssen Pharmaceutica, Piscataway, NJ)[208] acts by slowing intestinal motility and by affecting water and electrolyte movement through the bowel. Imodium inhibits peristaltic activity by a direct effect on the circular and longitudinal muscles of the intestinal wall. It is an excellent antidiarrheal agent for non-AIDS patients with mild to moderate diarrhea. Imodium is administered as follows:

Oral	1 to 2 capsules (2 mg/cap) orally every 6 hr prn
Nasointestinal feeding tube	10 to 20 cc (1 mg/cc) every 6 hr prn

Deodorized Tincture of Opium

Deodorized tincture of opium (DTO) (manufactured by Eli Lilly and Co., Indianapolis, Ind)[208] has an anticholinergic effect on gut peristalsis. It is an excellent antidiarrheal agent for non-AIDS patients with mild to moderate diarrhea. DTO is administered as follows:

Oral or nasointestinal feeding tube	15 to 20 gtt. every 4 to 6 hr prn

Sandostatin

Sandostatin (manufactured by Sandoz Pharmaceuticals Corp., East Hanover, NJ)[208] is a synthetic octapeptide with pharmacologic actions mimicking those of the natural hormone somatostatin.[103, 140] Sandostatin has the ability to suppress the secretion of serotonin,[140, 158, 173, 201, 270] vasoactive intestinal polypeptide,[32, 57, 152] gastrin,[10, 98, 229, 253, 270, 288] insulin,[73, 206, 267] glucagon,[5, 10, 37, 180] growth hormone, secretin, and pancreatic polypeptides.[55, 83, 158, 270, 288] It also exerts widespread effects on gastrointestinal function.[96, 202, 269, 270] It prolongs intestinal transit time, regulates intestinal water and electrolyte transport, and decreases splanchnic blood flow.*

Sandostatin differs from native somatostatin in four significant ways:

1. Sandostatin has a half-life of 60 to 112 minutes with a duration of action of 6 to 12 hours (somatostatin has a half-life of only 1 to 2 minutes).
2. Sandostatin can be administered subcutaneously or intravenously.
3. Sandostatin inhibits growth hormone secretion preferentially to insulin secretion.
4. Sandostatin is associated with less rebound hypersecretion when its effect tapers off.[140, 141]

Sandostatin is an excellent antidiarrheal agent for patients with diarrhea secondary to

1. Carcinoid tumor.
2. Pancreatic vasoactive polypeptide-secreting tumor (VI-Poma).
3. High-output ileostomy.

*References 60, 66, 71, 78, 133, 156, 190, 202, 218.

4. Short gut syndrome.
5. Enterocutaneous fistula.
6. Pancreatic fistula.
7. Inflammatory bowel disease.
8. AIDS enteropathy.

Diarrhea can be a life-threatening complication of AIDS. As many as 50% to 90% of all AIDS patients have gastrointestinal symptoms during the course of their disease. Diarrhea, usually chronic in nature and associated with weight loss and malnutrition, is the most common symptom.

The exact mechanism for the success of Sandostatin in the treatment of AIDS diarrhea is not well understood. Cook et al.[59] believe that the direct action of Sandostatin on the secretory apparatus of the gut controlled diarrhea in their patients. They also stated that this effect appeared to be mediated by the drug's suppressive action on intestinal transport rather than an effect on immunity. Because the AIDS virus is homologous to a vasoactive intestinal polypeptide (VIP) in its protein code amino acid sequences, Cook et al. have theorized that the AIDS virus may activate VIP receptors that induce the diarrheal response. Because Sandostatin is effective in controlling the secretory diarrhea associated with both AIDS and VIP-secreting tumors, it may be working at a membrane receptor that recognizes the VIP.

The majority of patients with AIDS with diarrhea who responded to Sandostatin therapy in the literature were infected with the coccidioidal protozoan, *Cryptosporidium*. This pathogen inhibits the microvillus border of the intestinal epithelial cells and is a common cause for severe, secretory diarrhea in immunosuppressed patients with AIDS. The clinical manifestations of this cryptosporidial infection include severe watery diarrhea, abdominal cramping, malabsorption, and weight loss. Since the diarrhea is refractory to conventional antidiarrheal therapy (e.g., Lomotil, Imodium, and DTO), patients frequently require hospitalization, intravenous fluids, and electrolyte replacement.

At present, most case reports indicate that Sandostatin can be successfully used to significantly reduce the volume of diarrhea in 30% to 40% of patients with AIDS with *Cryptosporidium*-induced secretory diarrhea.

Rene and associates[217] reported a significant reduction of stool output in two AIDS patients with isolated cryptosporidiosis following the subcutaneous administration of Sandostatin 100 μg twice daily.

Robinson and Fuegel[219] presented a case involving a man with AIDS-associated diarrhea without a demonstrable cryptosporidial infection. Sandostatin therapy was initiated at a dosage of 50 μg twice daily and eventually increased to three times daily. The patient's diarrhea rapidly ceased, his appetite improved, and he gained 9 kg in 6 weeks. Following 10 weeks of treatment, he had maintained his weight and experienced no further problems with diarrhea.

Fuessl et al.[95, 96] treated two patients with AIDS who had "uncontrollable diarrhea" with Sandostatin. The diarrhea was attributed to cytomegalovirus (CMV) enteritis. In these patients, Sandostatin therapy resulted in prompt improvement in both the frequency and volume of stools.

Further studies are clearly necessary to determine the role and mechanism of action of Sandostatin in the treatment of AIDS-related diarrhea. The preliminary reports from several ongoing clinical trials evaluating the effectiveness of Sandostatin in controlling AIDS diarrhea, however, are very encouraging.[59, 140, 141, 185, 219, 238]

ALBUMIN REPLACEMENT THERAPY
Therapeutic Indications

Patients with hypoalbuminemia (serum albumin <2.5 g%) have a decreased serum colloid osmotic pressure (COP) and bowel wall oncotic pressure (BWOP). Many nutritionists believe that a decreased serum COP and BWOP may cause delayed gastric emptying; decreased gut peristalsis; and reduced intestinal absorption of fluids, electrolytes and nutrients.* If the latter does occur, the patient will develop moderate to severe diarrhea and then gradually become malnourished. Because of the diarrhea, the patient's oral or nasointestinal enteral diet tolerance is compromised. If the abnormal serum COP and BWOP are not corrected, the patient will continue to have diarrhea, remain intolerant of both oral and nasointestinal enteral feedings, and will eventually require expensive parenteral diet therapy.

In view of this, many nutritionists attempt to correct the patient's serum COP and BWOP by intravenously administering 25% albumin or Hespan[208] (synthetic plasma expander) (see Calculation of Albumin Deficit, Albumin Administration, and Hespan Therapy). They believe that maximal oral or enteral diet

*References 9, 11, 12, 42–47, 67, 109, 192, 193, 278, 290.

tolerance is achieved when the patient's serum COP and BWOP are either equivalent to or greater than that associated with a serum albumin ≥2.5 g/dL. Unfortunately, the exact relationship between serum COP and BWOP and enteral diet tolerance has not been conclusively determined. Consequently, 25% albumin or Hespan replacement therapy remains controversial. At present, the author recommends replacement therapy only when treating patients with a serum albumin <2.5 g/dL who are candidates for either oral or nasointestinal enteral diet therapy.

Calculation of Albumin Deficit

The albumin deficit is calculated by means of the Andrassy formula:

$$AD = (DSA - ASA) \times 0.3 \times 10 \times wt. \ kg*$$

where, *AD* = albumin deficit, *DSA* = desired serum albumin (3 gm/dL), and *ASA* = actual serum albumin.

Albumin Administration

The albumin deficit is calculated per the Andrassy Formula. If the patient's serum albumin is <2.5g/dL, the deficit is replaced by administering 25% albumin, 25g intravenously every 4 to 6 hours. Once the deficit is replaced, the serum albumin level is rechecked. If it is ≥2.5g/dL, no further therapy is necessary. If the serum albumin is <2.5g/dL, the albumin deficit is recalculated and additional 25% albumin is administered until the serum albumin is ≥2.5g/dL.

HESPAN THERAPY

Characteristics

In view of the cost of albumin and the recent national shortage of it, many nutritionists are now administering inexpensive, readily available synthetic plasma expanders instead of albumin. Hespan (manufactured by Du Pont Pharmaceuticals, Wilmington, Del),[208] a synthetic plasma expander, has been successfully used for several years to increase the blood volume, serum COP, and BWOP of vascular, trauma, and surgical patients.† Consequently,

---

*Hardin T, Page C, Schwesinger W: Rapid replacement of serum albumin in patients receiving total parenteral nutrition. *Surg Gynecol Obstet* 1986; 163:359.

†References 101, 110, 162, 164, 169, 257, 272, 276.

TABLE 2-18.

Management of Enteral Nutrition–Induced Physiologic and Metabolic Complications

Complication	Treatment

Diarrhea	1. Check the actual serum albumin (ASA) level. If the ASA level <2.5 g%, calculate the albumin deficit (AD) per the Andrassy Formula:
	
	$$AD = (2.5 - ASA) \times 0.3 \times 10 \times wt\ kg$$
	
	Then administer 25% albumin 25 g intravenously q 6 hr until the calculated albumin deficit is replaced. Recheck the serum albumin. If the serum albumin level ≥2.5 g%, no further albumin therapy is necessary. If the level <2.5 g%, recalculate the albumin deficit and administer additional albumin intravenously until the serum albumin ≥2.5 g%.
	
	2. Administer antidiarrheal agents:
	    Deodorized Tincture of Opium (DTO) 15–20 qtts po or per nasointestinal tube q 4–6 hr prn
	    or
	    Lomotil 1–2 caps (2.5 mg/tab) po q 4–6 hr or 5–10 cc (2.5 mg/5 cc) per nasointestinal tube q 4–6 hr prn
	    or
	    Imodium 1–2 caps (2 mg/cap) po q 4–6 hr or 10–20 cc (1 mg/5 cc) per nasointestinal tube q 4–6 hr prn
	    or
	    Sandostatin 50–300 μg subcutaneously or intravenously q 6 hr prn for diarrhea
	
	3. If 1 and 2 fail to treat the diarrhea, discontinue the current enteral diet and begin Compleat Modified Formula (full strength) enteral diet at 40 cc/hr per pump. If tolerated (no diarrhea), then increase the infusion rate per the Isosomolar Enteral Diet Infusion Schedule.
	
	4. If 1, 2, and 3 fail, discontinue enteral nutritional therapy and begin parenteral nutritional therapy.

Residuals (>150 cc)	1. Examine the patient and rule out the possibility of either a mechanical intestinal obstruction or paralytic ileus.
	2. Confirm the position of the feeding tube in the small bowel per KUB.
	3. Check the serum potassium and calcium levels.
	4. Consider a pharmacologic etiology.
Hyperglycemia (>160 mg/dL)	Reduce the oral glucose intake and administer regular insulin subcutaneously per a sliding scale regimen. If this fails to maintain the serum glucose ≤160 mg%, discontinue the current full-strength enteral diet and begin either a less concentrated infusion of the current diet or begin a new full-strength diet which has a lower glucose content (consult the *Physicians' Desk Reference [PDR]*) at the previous infusion rate.
Hypoglycemia (<70 mg/dL)	Administer (immediately) one ampule of $D_{50}W$ intravenously and then recheck the serum glucose. If the serum glucose remains <70 mg%, administer additional intravenous $D_{50}W$ until the serum glucose ≥70 mg%. If the patient continues to require intravenous glucose supplements, discontinue the current full-strength enteral diet and begin a new full-strength diet which has a greater glucose content (consult the *PDR*) at the previous infusion rate.
Hypernatremia (>145 mEq/L)	Reduce or discontinue all oral and intravenous sodium intake. If this fails to maintain the serum sodium ≤145 mEq/L, discontinue the current full-strength enteral diet and begin either a less concentrated infusion of the current diet or begin a new full-strength diet which has a lower sodium content (consult the *PDR*) at the previous infusion rate.
Hyponatremia (<135 mEq/L)	Administer additional sodium intravenously until the serum sodium ≥135 mEq/L. If intravenous sodium supplementation fails to correct the hyponatremia, discontinue the full-strength enteral diet and begin a new full-strength diet which has a greater sodium content (consult the *PDR*) at the previous infusion rate.

Continued.

TABLE 2–18 (cont.).

Complication	Treatment
Hyperkalemia (>5 mEq/L)	Discontinue all oral and intravenous potassium intake. If this fails to maintain the serum potassium ≤5 mEq/L, discontinue the current full-strength enteral diet and begin a new full-strength diet which has a lower potassium content (consult the *PDR*) at the previous infusion rate.
Hypokalemia (<3.5 mEq/L)	Administer additional potassium orally or intravenously until the serum potassium ≥3.5 mEq/L. If the patient continues to require excessive oral or intravenous potassium supplements, discontinue the current full-strength enteral diet and begin a new full-strength diet which has a greater potassium content (consult the *DR*) at the previous infusion rate.
Hyperphosphatemia (>4.5 mEq/L)	Discontinue all oral and intravenous phosphate intake. If this fails to maintain the serum phosphate ≥4.5 mEq/L, discontinue the current full-strength enteral diet and begin a new full-strength diet which has a lower phosphate content (consult the *PDR*) at the previous infusion rate.
Hypophosphatemia (<2.5 mg/dL)	Administer additional phosphate either orally as Neutra-Phos 1–2 caps (250 mg/cap) dissolved in 75–150 cc of tube feeding 2–4 times daily (consult the *PDR* for additional enteral phosphate preparations) or intravenously as sodium or potassium phosphate to maintain the serum phosphate ≥2.5 mg%. NOTE: **The daily intravenous phosphate dosage should not exceed 60 mM.**
Hypermagnesemia (>2.7 mg/dL)	Discontinue all intravenous and oral magnesium intake. If this fails to maintain the serum magnesium ≤2.7 mg%, discontinue the current full-strength enteral diet and begin a new full-strength diet which has a lower magnesium content (consult the *PDR*) at the previous infusion rate.

Hypomagnesemia (<1.6 mg/dL)	Administer additional magnesium either orally or intravenously to maintain the serum magnesium ≥1.6 mg%. Consult the *PDR* for the various enteral and parenteral magnesium preparations.
Hypercalcemia (>10.5 mg/dL)	Discontinue all oral and intravenous calcium supplements. If this fails to maintain the serum calcium ≤10.5 mg%, discontinue the current full-strength enteral diet and begin a new full-strength diet which has a lower calcium content (consult the *PDR*) at the previous infusion rate.
Hypocalcemia (<8.5 mg/dL)	Administer additional calcium either orally as Titralac 2 tsp added to the tube feeding bid or intravenously as Calcium Gluceptate 10–30 mEq daily to maintain the serum calcium ≥8.5 mg%. Consult the *PDR* for additional enteral and parenteral calcium preparations.
High serum zinc (>150 µg/dL)	Discontinue all oral and intravenous zinc intake until the serum zinc ≤150 mcg%.
Low serum zinc (<55 µg/dL)	Administer additional zinc either orally as zinc sulfate 200 mg tid or qid or intravenously as elemental zinc 2–5 mg daily to maintain a serum zinc ≥55 mcg%. Consult the *PDR* for additional enteral and parenteral zinc preparations.
High serum copper (>140 µg/dL)	Discontinue all oral and intravenous copper intake until the serum copper ≤140 mcg%.
Low serum copper (<70 µg/dL)	Administer additional copper either orally (consult the *PDR* for the various enteral copper preparations) or intravenously as elemental copper 2–5 mg daily to maintain a serum copper >70 mcg%.

the author believes that Hespan could also be effectively used as an alternative to albumin replacement therapy when treating patients with a serum albumin <2.5g/dL who require oral or enteral diet therapy.

Dosage

Patients with a serum albumin <2.5g/dL and subsequently a low serum COP and BWOP are initially treated with Hespan, 250 cc intravenously. The dosage is then repeated after 24 hours if (1) the patient's serum COP and BWOP remain low and the enteral diet is not tolerated *and* (2) the patient has no cardiovascular problems that would prohibit additional therapy. At present, the exact therapeutic dosage of Hespan has not been determined. One hopes that, in the near future, well-designed clinical trials will determine the exact therapeutic dosage of Hespan and confirm its role in enteral diet therapy.

PHYSIOLOGIC AND METABOLIC COMPLICATIONS

Enterally fed patients may develop physiologic and metabolic complications secondary to the therapy. Table 2–18 lists several of these complications and briefly discusses their management.

REFERENCES

1. Adams S, et al: Enteral versus parenteral nutritional support following laparotomy for trauma: A randomized prospective trial. *J Trauma* 1986; 10:882–891.
2. Adrawi MSM, Newsholme EA: Glutamine metabolism in lymphocytes of the rat. *Biochem J* 1982; 208:743.
3. Alexander JW, et al: Nutritional immuno-modulators in burn patients. *Crit Care Med* 1990; 18:S149–S153.
4. Alexander JW, et al: The importance of lipid type in the diet after burn injury. *Ann Surg* 1986; 204:1–8.
5. Altimari AF, et al: Use of somatostatin analogue (SMS 210-995) in the glucagonoma syndrome. *Surgery* 1986; 100:989–996.
6. Alverdy J, Aoys E, Moss G: Total parenteral nutrition promotes bacterial translocation from the gut. *Surgery* 1988; 104:185.
7. American Medical Association, Department of Foods and

Nutrition's Guidelines for Essential Trace Element Preparations for Parenteral Use. A statement of the Nutritional Advisory Group. *JPEN* 1979; 8:263–267.

8. American Medical Association, Department of Foods and Nutrition Expert Panel for Nutrition Advisory Group. Guidelines for essential trace element preparations for parenteral use. *JAMA* 1979; 241:241.

9. Anderson BJ: Tube feeding: Is diarrhea inevitable? *Am J Nurs* 1986; 704–706.

10. Anderson JV, Bloom SR: Neuroendocrine tumors of the gut: Long-term therapy with the somatostatin analogue SMS 201-995. *Scand J Gastroenterol* 1986; 21(suppl 119):115–128.

11. Andrassy RJ: Enteral elemental nutrition in pediatric surgery. *Contemp Surg* 1986; 28(suppl 4A).

12. Andrassy RJ: Enteral elemental nutrition in pediatric surgery. *Contemp Surg* 1985; 28:24–29.

13. Armstrong MD, Stave U: A study of plasma free amino acid levels. A study of factors affecting validity of amino acid analysis. *Metabolism* 1973; 22:549.

14. Askanazi J, et al: Muscle and plasma amino acids following injury: Influence of intercurrent infection. *Ann Surg* 1980; 192:78.

15. Askanazi J, et al: Muscle and plasma amino acids after injury: Hypocaloric glucose vs. amino acid infusion. *Ann Surg* 1980; 191:465.

16. Askanazi J, et al: Nutrition and the respiratory system. *Crit Care Med* 1982; 10:163–172.

17. A.S.P.E.N. Board of Directors. Guidelines for the use of enteral nutrition in adult patients. *JPEN* 1987; 11:435–439.

18. Babayan VK: Early history and preparation of MCT, in *Zeitschrift fur Ernahrungs-wisenschaft* Supplementa 17. Darmstadt: Dr. Dietrich Steinkopf, 1974.

19. Babayan VK: Medium-chain triglycerides and structured lipids. *Lipids* 1987; 22:47.

20. Babayan VK: Medium-chain length fatty acid esters and their medical and nutritional applications (abst). *J Am Oil Chem Soc* 1981; 58:49A–51A.

21. Babayan VK: Medium-chain triglycerides: Their composition, preparation and application. *J Am Oil Chem Soc* 1967; 45:23–25.

22. Bach AC, Babayan VK: Medium chain triglycerides: An update. *Am J Clin Nutr* 1982; 36:950–962.

23. Baker JP, Lemoyne M: Nutritional support in the critically ill patient: If, when, how and what? *Crit Care Clin* 1987; 3:97–113.

24. Barbul A, et al: Arginine stimulates lymphocyte immune response in healthy human beings. *Surgery* 1981; 90:244–251.

25. Barden RP, et al: The influence of the serum protein on the motility of the small intestine. *Surgery* 1979; 86:307–315.

26. Bassilli RH: Nutritional support in long term intensive care with special reference to ventilator patients: A review. *Can Anaesth Soc J* 1981; 28:17–21.

27. Begin ME, Das UN: A deficiency in dietary gamma-linolenic and/or eicosapentaenoic acids may determine individual susceptibility to AIDS. *Med Hypotheses* 1986; 20:1–8.

28. Beisel WR: Metabolic response to infection, in Kinney J, Jeejeebhoy K, Hill G, et al (eds): *Nutrition and Metabolism in Patient Care*. Philadelphia: WB Saunders Co/Harcourt Brace Jovanovich, 1988, p 605.

29. Beisel WR, et al: Single-nutrient effects on immunologic functions. *JAMA* 1981; 245:53–58.

30. Bell SJ, Wyatt J: Nutritional guidelines for burned patients. *J Am Diet Assoc* 1986; 86:648–653.

31. Bell SJ, et al: Osmolality of beverages commonly provided on clear and full liquid menu. *Nutr Clin Prac,* in press.

32. Benson W, et al: Control of watery diarrhea syndrome in a patient with vasoactive intestinal polypeptide-secreting tumor, using SMS 201-995 and dexamethasone. *Scand J Gastroenterol* 1986; 21(suppl 119):107–116.

33. Bergstrom J, et al: Intracellular free amino acid concentration in human muscle tissue. *J Appl Physiol* 1974; 36:643.

34. Beyer PO, Frankenfield DC: Enteral nutrition in extreme short bowel. *Nutr Clin Pract* 1987; 2:60–64.

35. Blackburn GL, et al: Branched chain amino acid administration and metabolism during starvation, injury and infection. *Surgery* 1979; 86:307–315.

36. Blackburn GL, et al: Enteral tube feeding: State of the art. *J Gastroenterol* 1985; 23:7–15.

37. Boden G, et al: Treatment of inoperable glucagonoma with

the long-acting somatostatin analogue SMS 201-995. *N Engl J Med* 1986; 314:1686–1689.

38. Border JR, et al: The gut origin septic states in blunt multiple trauma (ISS-40) in the ICU. *Ann Surg* 1987; 206:427–448.

39. Bower RH, et al: Branched chain amino acid enriched solution in the septic patient. *Ann Surg* 1986; 203:13–20.

40. Bower RH, et al: Postoperative enteral vs. parenteral nutrition. *Arch Surg* 1986; 121:1040–1045.

41. Brennan MF, et al: Report of a research workshop: Branched-chain amino acids in stress and injury. *JPEN* 1986; 10:446–452.

42. Brinson RR: Hypoalbuminemia, diarrhea and the acquired immunodeficiency syndrome. *Ann Intern Med* 1985; 102:413.

43. Brinson RR, Curtis WD, Singh M: Diarrhea in the intensive care unit. The role of hypoalbuminemia and the response to a peptide-based diet. *J Am Coll Nutr* 1987; 15:506.

44. Brinson RR, Kolts B: Hypoalbuminemia as an indicator of diarrheal incidence in critically ill patient. *Crit Care Med* 1987; 15:506–509.

45. Brinson RR, et al: Diarrhea in the intensive care unit: The role of hypoalbuminemia and the response to a clinically defined diet (case reports and review of the literature). *J Am Coll Nutr* 1987; 6:517–522.

46. Brinson RR, et al: Hypoalbuminemia-associated diarrhea in critically ill patients. *J Crit Ill* Sept 1987.

47. Brinson RR, et al: Intestinal absorption of peptide enteral formulas in hypoproteinemic (volume expanded) rats: A paired analysis. *Crit Care Med* 1989; 17:657–660.

48. Burch RE, Hahn HKJ: Trace elements in human nutrition. *Med Clin North Am* 1979; 63:1057–1068.

49. Catali-Batcner EL, et al: Complications occurring during enteral nutrition support: A prospective study. *JPEN* 1983; 7:546–552.

50. Cello JP, et al: Controlled clinical trial of octreotide for refractory AIDS-associated diarrhea. Abstract 163 presented at the American Digestive Week Meeting, San Antonio, Tex, May 1990.

51. Cerra FB, et al: A multicenter trial of branched chain en-

riched amino acid infusion (FO8O) in hepatic encephalopathy (HE). *JPEN* 1985; 9:288.

52. Cerra FB, et al: Branched chain metabolic support: A prospective, randomized, double blind trial in surgical stress. *Ann Surg* 1984; 199:286–291.

53. Cerra FB, et al: Branched chains support postoperative protein synthesis. *Surgery* 1982; 92:192–199.

54. Cerra FB, et al: Nitrogen retention in critically ill patients in proportion to the branched chain amino acid load. *Crit Care Med* 1983; 11:775–778.

55. Ch'ng JL, et al: Remission of symptoms during long-term treatment of metastatic pancreatic endocrine tumors with long-acting somatostatin analogue. *Br J Med* 1985; 2:981–982.

56. Chua B, et al: Effect of leucine and metabolites of branched chain amino acids on protein turnover in heart. *J Biol Chem* 1979; 254:8358–8362.

57. Clements D, et al: Regression of metastatic VIPoma with somatostatin analogue SMS 201-295. *Lancet* 1985; 1:874–875.

58. Cobb JM, Cartmill AM, Gilsdorf RB: Early postoperative nutritional support using the serosal tunnel jejunostomy. *JPEN* 1981; 5:397–401.

59. Cook DJ, et al: Somatostatin treatment for cryptosporidial diarrhea in a patient with acquired immunodeficiency syndrome (AIDS). *Ann Intern Med* 1988; 108:708–709.

60. Cooper JC, et al: Effects of a long-acting somatostatin analogue in patients with severe ileostomy diarrhea. *Br J Surg* 1986; 73:128–131.

61. Cotzias GC: *Trace Subst. Environ. Health.* Proc. Mo 1st Annual Conference. 1967, p 5.

62. Council on Scientific Affairs, American Medical Association. American Medical Association concepts of nutrition and health. *JAMA* 1979; 242:2335–2338.

63. Cutie AJ, Altman E, Lenkel L: Compatibility of enteral products with commonly employed drug additives. *JPEN* 1983; 7:186–191.

64. Daly JM, et al: Immune and metabolic effects of arginine in the surgical patient. *Ann Surg* 1988; 208:512–522.

65. Deitch EA, Winterton J, Berg R: Effect of starvation, malnutrition and trauma on the gastrointestinal tract flora and bacterial translocation. *Arch Surg* 1987; 122:1019–1024.

66. Dharmsathaphorn K, et al: Somatostatin decreases diarrhea in patients with short bowel syndrome. *J Clin Gastroenterol* 1982; 4:521–524.

67. Diamond JM: Osmotic water flow in leaky epithelia. *J Membr Biol* 1979; 5:195–216.

68. Dominioni L, et al: Enteral feeding in burn hypermetabolism: Nutritional and metabolic effects of different levels of caloric and protein intake. *JPEN* 1985; 9:269–279.

69. Dominioni L, et al: Nitrogen balance and liver changes in burned guinea pigs undergoing prolonged high protein enteral feeding. *Surg Forum* 1983; 34:99–101.

70. Duel HJ, Jr: *The Lipids, Their Chemistry and Biochemistry,* vols 1–3. New York: Interscience Publishers, 1957.

71. Dueno MI, et al: Effect of somatostatin analogue on water and electrolyte transport and transit time in human small bowel. *Dig Dis Sci* 1987; 32:1092–1096.

72. Dworkin BM, et al: Selenium deficiency in the acquired immunodeficiency syndrome. *JPEN* 1986; 10:405–407.

73. Ellison EC, et al: Modulation of functional gastrointestinal endocrine tumors by endogenous and exogenous somatostatin. *Am J Surg* 1986; 151:668–675.

74. Esvelt BM, et al: *Handbook of Enteral Nutrition.* El Segundo, Calif: Medical Specifics Publishing, 1983.

75. Fairclough PD, et al: A comparison of the absorption of two protein hydrolysates and their effects on water and electrolyte movements in the human jejunum. *Gut* 1980; 21:829.

76. Fairclough PD, et al: New evidence for intact di- and tripeptide absorption. *Gut* 1975; 16:843a.

77. Fanslow KC, et al: Effect of nucleotide restriction and supplementation on resistance to experimental nurine candidiasis. *JPEN* 1988; 12:49–52.

78. Fedorak RN, Field M: Antidiarrheal therapy. Prospects for new agents. *Dig Dis Sci* 1987; 32:192–205.

79. Felig P: Amino acid metabolism in man. *Annu Rev Biochem* 1975; 44:933.

80. Felig P, Wahren J, Raf L: Evidence of inter-organ amino-acid transport by blood cells in humans. *Proc Natl Acad Sci USA* 1973; 70:1775–1779.

81. Fell GS, Halls D, Shenkin A: in Shapcott D, Hubert J

(eds): *Chromium in Nutrition and Metabolism.* New York: Elsevier North-Holland, 1979, pp 105–111.

82. Fiaccadori F, et al: Branched chain amino acid enriched solutions in the treatment of hepatic encephalopathy: A controlled trial, in Capocaccia L, Fischer JE, et al (eds): *Hepatic Encephalopathy in Chronic Liver Failure.* New York: Plenum Publishing Corp, 1984, pp 325–334.

83. Fiasse R, et al: Short-term effects of the long-acting soma-tostatin analogue SMS 201-995 in five cases of APUDoma (four with metastases) and in one case of systemic macro-cytosis. *Scand J Gastroenterol* 1986; 21(suppl 119):212–216.

84. Finch CA, Huebers H: Perspectives in iron metabolism. *N Engl J Med* 1982; 306:1520–1528.

85. *Foods, Fats and Oils,* ed 5. Washington, DC: Institute of Shortening and Edible Oils, 1982.

86. Ford EG, Andrassy RJ: Serum albumin (oncotic pressure) correlates with enteral feeding tolerance in the pediatric surgical patient. *J Pediatr Surg* 1987; 22:597–599.

87. Fox AD, et al: Reduction of the severity of enterocolitis by glutamine supplemented enteral diets. *Surg Forum* 1987; 38:43.

88. Frank HA, Green LC: Successful use of a bulk laxative to control the diarrhea of tube feeding. *Scand J Plast Reconstr Surg* 1977; 13:193–194.

89. Freed BA, et al: Enteral nutrition: Frequency of formula modification. *JPEN* 1981; 5:40.

90. Freedman Z, Marks KH, Maisels J: Effect of parenteral fat emulsions on pulmonary reticuloendothelial systems in the newborn infant. *Pediatrics* 1978; 61:694.

91. Freund H, Atamian S, Fischer JE: Chromium deficiency during total parenteral nutrition. *JAMA* 1979; 241:496–497.

92. Freund H, Fischer JE: Nitrogen conserving quality of the branched chain amino acids: Possible regulator effect of valine in postinjury muscle catabolism. *Surg Forum* 1978; 29:69–72.

93. Freund H, Fischer JE: The use of branched chain amino acids (BCAA) in acute hepatic encephalopathy. *Clin Nutr* 1986; 5:135–138.

94. Freund H, Yoshimura N, Fischer JE: The effect of branched chain amino acids and hypertonic glucose infu-

sions on post-injury catabolism in the rat. *Surgery* 1980; 87:401–408.

95. Fuessl HS, et al: Effects of a long-acting somatostatin analogue (SMS 201-995) on postprandial gastric emptying of Tc-tin colloid and mouth-to-caecum transit time in man. *Digestion* 1987; 36:101–107.

96. Fuessl HS, et al: Symptomatic treatment of uncontrollable diarrhea in AIDS with the somatostatin analog SMS 201-995. *Klin Wochenschr* 1988; 66(suppl 13):240–241.

97. Fuessl HS, et al: Treatment of secretory diarrhea in AIDS with the somatostatin analog SMS 201-295. *Klin Wochenschr* 1989; 67:452–455.

98. Geelhoed GW, et al: Somatostatin analogue: Effects on hypergastrinemia and hypercalcitoninemia. *Surgery* 1986; 100:962–970.

99. Gimmon Z, Freund HR, Fischer JE: The optimal branched chain amino acid ratio in the injury-adapted amino acid formulation. *JPEN* 1985; 9:133.

100. Goldman DW, Pickett WC, Goetzl EJ: Human neutrophil chemotactic and degranulating activities of leukotriene B5 derived from eicosapentaenoic acid. *Biochem Biophys Res Commun* 1983; 117:282.

101. Goldsmith GA: Trace element regulation of immunity and infection. *J Am Coll Nutr* 1985; 51:727–733.

102. Gollub S, Vanichanan C, Schaefer, et al: A study of safer plasma substitutes. *Surg Gynecol Obstet* 1969; 128:1235.

103. Goodman AG, Gilman L: *The Pharmacological Basis of Therapeutics,* ed 7. New York: Macmillan Publishing Co, 1985.

104. Granger DN, Brinson RR: Intestinal absorption of elemental and standard enteral formulas in hypoproteinemic (volume expanded) rats. *JPEN* 1988; 12:278.

105. Green ML, Harry J: *Nutrition in Contemporary Nursing Practice*. New York, John Wiley & Sons, 1981.

106. Greenberger NJ, Skillman TG: Medium chain triglycerides. *N Engl J Med* 1969; 230:1045–1058.

107. Guisard DG: Metabolic effects of a medium chain triglyceride emulsion injected intravenously in man. *Horm Metab Res* 1972; 4:509.

108. Hamawy KJ, et al: The effect of lipid emulsions on reticuloendothelial system function in the injured animal. *JPEN* 1985; 9:559.

109. Hardin TC, Page CP, Schweisinger WH: Rapid replacement of serum albumin in patients receiving total parenteral nutrition. *Surg Gynecol Obstet* 1986; 163:359–362.

110. Haupt MT, Rackow EC: Colloid osmotic pressure and fluid resuscitation with hetastarch, albumin, and saline. *Crit Care Med* 1982; 10:159.

111. Hegarty JE, et al: Effects of concentration on in vivo absorption of a peptide containing protein hydrolysate. *Gut* 1982; 23:304.

112. Herbert V: The nutritional anemias. *Hosp Pract* 1980; 12:65–69.

113. Herman-Zaidins MG: Malabsorption in adults: Etiology, evaluation and management. *J Am Diet Assoc* 1986; 86:1171–1181.

114. Heymsfield SB: Metabolic changes associated with refeeding. *A.S.P.E.N. Update* 1982; 4:1–2.

115. Heymsfield SB, et al: Cardiac abnormalities in cachectic patients before and during nutritional repletion. *Am Heart J* 1987; 95:584.

116. Hickey MS, Weaver KE: Enteral nutrition, in Luce J, Pierson D (eds): *Critical Care Medicine.* Philadelphia, WB Saunders Co, 1988, pp 355–382.

117. Hiebert JM, et al: Comparison of continuous vs. intermittent tube feedings in adult burn patients. *JPEN* 1980; 5:73–75.

118. Hilditch TP, Williams PN: *The Chemical Constitution of Natural Fats,* ed 4. New York: John Wiley & Sons, 1964.

119. Hindale JG, Lipkowitz GS, et al: Prolonged enteral nutrition in malnourished patients with nonelemental feeding. Reappraisal of surgical technique, safety and costs. *Am J Surg* 1985; 149:334–338.

120. Holtz L, Milton J, Sturek JK: Compatibility of medications with enteral feedings. *JPEN* 1987; 11:183–186.

121. Hoover HC, et al: Nutritional benefits of immediate postoperative jejunal feeding of an elemental diet. *Am J Surg* 1980; 139:153–158.

122. Howard PA, Hannaman KN: Warfarin resistance linked to enteral nutrition products. *J Am Diet Assoc* 1985; 85:713–714.

123. Hull S: Enteral versus parenteral nutrition support rationale for increased use of enteral feeding. *J Gastroenterol* 1985; 23:55–63.

124. Husami T, Abumrad NN: Adverse metabolic consequences of nutritional support: Micronutrients. *Surg Clin North Am* 1986; 66:1049–1069.

125. Hutson SM, Cree RC, Harper AE: Regulation of leucine and aketoisocaproic acid metabolism in skeletal muscle. *J Biochem* 1980; 255:2418–2426.

126. Hwang TL, et al: Preservation of small bowel mucosa using glutamine enriched parenteral nutrition. *Surg Forum* 1987; 38:56.

127. Inoue S, et al: Increased gut blood flow with early enteral feeding in burned guinea pigs, in press.

128. Inoue S, et al: Is glutamine beneficial in postburn nutritional support? *Curr Surg* 1988; 45:110–113.

129. Inoue S, et al: Prevention of yeast translocation across the gut by a single enteral feeding after burn injury. *JPEN* 1989; 13:565–567.

130. Ireton-Jones CS, Turner NW: The use of respiratory quotient to determine the efficacy of nutrition support regimens. *J Am Diet Assoc* 1983; 82:117–123.

131. Jacobs S, Wester PO: Balance study of twenty trace elements during total parenteral nutrition in man. *Br J Nutr* 1977; 37:107.

132. Jacobson E, et al: Combined effects of glutamine and epidermal growth factors (ECF) on GI mucosal cellularity. *Surgery* 1988; 104:358.

133. Jaros W, et al: Successful treatment of idiopathic secretory diarrhea of infancy with the somatostatin analogue SMS 201-995. *Gastroenterology* 1988; 94:189–193.

134. Jeejeebhoy KN, et al: Chromium deficiency, glucose intolerance and neuropathy reversed by chromium supplementation in a patient receiving long term total parenteral nutrition. *Am J Clin Nutr* 1977; 30:531.

135. Johnson DJ, et al: Branched chain amino acid supplementation fails to reduce posttraumatic protein catabolism. *Surg Forum* 1984; 35:102.

136. Jones BJ, Payne S, Silk DBA: Indications for pump-assisted enteral feeding. *Lancet* 1980; 1:1057–1058.

137. Kaiser MH: Medium-chain triglycerides. *Adv Intern Med* 1971; 17:301–322.

138. Kapadia CR, et al: Alterations in glutamine metabolism in response to operative stress and food deprivation. *Surg Forum* 1982; 33:19.

139. Kapadia CR, et al: Maintenance of skeletal muscle intracellular glutamine during standard surgical trauma. *JPEN* 1985; 9:583–589.

140. Katz MD, Erstad B: Octreotide, a new somatostatin analogue. *Clin Pharm* 1989; 8:225–273.

141. Katz MD, et al: Treatment of severe cryptosporidium-related diarrhea with octreotide in a patient with AIDS. *Drug Intell Clin Pharm* 1988; 22:134–136.

142. Kaunitz H: Clinical uses of medium-chain triglycerides. *Drug Ther* 1978; 91–99.

143. Kause A: Parenteral and enteral nutrition of the thermally injured patient. *Ann Chir Gynaecol* 1980; 69:197–201.

144. Kay RM, et al: Elemental and liquid diets in surgery, in Deitel M (ed): *Nutrition in Clinical Surgery*. Baltimore: Williams & Wilkins Co, 1980, pp 29–41.

145. Keohane PP, et al: Relation between osmolality of diet and gastrointestinal side effects in enteral nutrition. *Br Med J* 1984; 288:573–680.

146. Reference deleted in proofs.

147. Keohane PP, et al: The roles of lactose and *Clostridium difficile* in the pathogenesis of enteral feeding associated diarrhea. *Clin Nutr* 1983; 1:246–259.

148. Khalidi N: Trace elements: An update. *Nutr Suppl Serv* 1988; 8.

149. Kien EL, Ganthor HZ: Manifestations of chronic selenium deficiency in a child receiving total parenteral nutrition. *Am J Clin Nutr* 1984; 37:319–321.

150. Kinney JM, Felig P: The metabolic response to injury and infection, in Degroot LJ, Cahill GF (eds): *Endocrinology*, vol 3. New York, 1989, Grune & Stratton.

151. Kinney JM, et al: Influence of nutrients on ventilation. *Rev Clin Nutr* 1984; 54:921–923.

152. Koelz A, et al: Escape of response to a long-acting somatostatin analogue (SMS 201-995) in patients with VIPoma. *Gastroenterology* 1987; 92:527–531.

153. Koruda MJ, et al: Enteral nutrition in the critically ill. *Crit Care Clin* 1987; 1:133–135.

154. Kotler DP: Diarrhea in AIDS—diagnosis and management. *Res Staff Phys* 1987; 33:30–41.

155. Kovacevic Z, McGivan JD: Mitochondrial metabolism of glutamine and glutamate and its physiologic significance. *Physiol Rev* 1983; 63:547.

156. Krejs GJ, Browne R, Raskin P: Effect of intravenous somatostatin on jejunal absorption of glucose, amino acids, water and electrolytes. *Gastroenterology* 1980; 78:26–31.

157. Kulkarni AD, et al: Influence of dietary nucleotide restriction on bacterial sepsis and phagocytic cell function in mice. *Arch Surg* 1986; 121:169–172.

158. Kvols LK, et al: The treatment of metastatic islet cell carcinoma with a somatostatin analogue (SMS 201-995). *Ann Intern Med* 1987; 107:162–168.

159. Kvols LK, et al: The treatment of the malignant carcinoid syndrome—evaluation of a long-acting somatostatin analogue. *N Engl J Med* 1986; 315:663–666.

160. Larkin JM, Maylan JA: Complete enteral support of thermally ill patients. *Am J Surg* 1976; 131:722–724.

161. Lauser ME, Saba TM: Neutrophil mediated lung location of bacteria: A mechanism for pulmonary injury. *Surgery* 1982; 90:473.

162. Lazrove S, Waxman K, Shippy C, et al: Hemodynamic, blood volume, and oxygen transport responses to albumin and hydroxyethyl starch infusions in critically ill postoperative patients. *Crit Care Med* 1989; 8:302.

163. Lee TH, et al: Effect of dietary enrichment with eicosapentaenoic acids in vitro neutrophil and monocyte leukotriene generation and neutrophil function. *N Engl J Med* 1985; 312:1217.

164. Lee WH, Cooper N, Weidner MG, et al: Clinical evaluation of a new plasma expander: Hydroxyethyl starch. *J Trauma* 1968; 8:381.

165. Li JB, Lefferson LS: Influence of amino acid availability on protein turnover in perfused skeletal muscle. *Biochem Biophys Acta* 1978; 544:351–359.

166. Lochs H, et al: Is tube feeding with elemental diets a primary therapy of Crohn's disease? *Klin Wochenschr* 1981; 62:821–825.

167. Lokesh BR, Hsieh HL, Kinsella JE: Peritoneal macrophage from mice fed dietary (w3) polyunsaturated fatty acids secrete low levels of prostaglandins. *J Nutr* 1986; 116:2547.

168. Love AHG: Metabolic response to malnutrition: Its relevance to enteral feeding. *Gut* 1986; 27(suppl S1):9–13.

169. Lucus EC, Weaver D, Higgins RF, et al: Effects of albumin versus nonalbumin resuscitation on plasma volume and renal excretory function. *J Trauma* 1978; 18:564.

170. Maejima K, Deitch E, Berg R: Promotion by burn stress of the translocation of bacteria from the gastrointestinal tracts of mice. *Arch Surg* 1984; 119:166–172.

171. Magrum LJ, Johnstone PV: Effect of culture in vitro with eicosatetraenoic and eicosapentaenoic acids in fatty acid composition, prostaglandin synthesis and chemiluminescence of rat peritoneal macrophages. *Biochem Biophys Acta* 1984; 836:354.

172. Mamal JJ: Percutaneous endoscopic gastrostomy. *Nutr Clin Pract* 1987; 2:65–75.

173. March HM, et al: Carcinoid crisis during anesthesia: Successful treatment with a somatostatin analogue. *Anesthesiology* 1987; 66:89–91.

174. Marshall JC, et al: The microbiology of multiple organ failure. *Arch Surg* 1988; 123:309–315.

175. Martin BK, Slingerland AW, Jenks JS: Severe hypophosphatemia associated with nutritional support. *Nutr Suppl Serv* 1985; 5:34–38.

176. Mascioli EA, Bistrian BR, Babayan VK: Medium chain triglycerides and structured lipids as unique nonglucose energy sources in hyperalimentation. *Lipids* 1987; 22:421.

177. Mascioli EA, et al: Effect of a menhaden oil diet on survival to endotoxin in guinea pigs. *Am J Clin Nutr,* in press.

178. Mascioli EA, et al: Endotoxin challenge after menhaden oil diet: Effects on survival of guinea pigs. *Am J Clin Nutr* 1989; 49:277–282.

179. Mascioli EA, et al: Enhanced survival to endotoxin in guinea pigs fed i.v. fish oil. *Lipids* 1989; 23:623–625.

180. Maton PN, et al: Use of somatostatin and somatostatin analogues in a patient with glucagonoma. *J Clin Endocrinol Metab* 1981; 53:543–549.

181. McClain CJ: Trace metal abnormalities in adults during hyperalimentation. *JPEN* 1981; 5:424–429.

182. Mecray PM, Barden RP, Ravdin IS: Nutritional edema: Its effect on gastric emptying time before and after gastric operations. *Surgery* 1937; 1:53.

183. Meisel JL, et al: Overwhelming watery diarrhea associated with cryptosporidium in an immunosuppressed patient. *Gastroenterology* 1975; 70:1156–1160.

184. Mequid MM, et al: Effect of enteral diet on albumin and

ureasynthesis: Comparison with partially hydrolyzed protein diet. *J Surg Res* 1981; 37:16–24.

185. Mercure L, et al: Inhibition of the AIDS virus replication by a long-acting somatostatin analog. Presented at the 4th International Conference on AIDS, Stockholm, June 12–16, 1988, Book II, p. 153, Abstr no. 3548.

186. Miller RM, et al: Skeletal changes of copper deficiency in infants receiving prolonged total parenteral nutritional. *J Pediatr* 1980; 92:947–949.

187. Mochizuki H, et al: Effect of diet rich in branched chain amino acids on severely burned guinea pigs. *J Trauma* 1986; 26:1077–1085.

188. Mochizuki H, et al: Mechanism of prevention of postburn hypermetabolism and catabolism by early enteral feeding. *Ann Surg* 1984; 200:297–310.

189. Mochizuki H, et al: Nitrogen balance and liver changes in burned guinea pigs undergoing prolonged high protein enteral feedings. *Surg Forum* 1983; 34:99–101.

190. Moller N, et al: Effects of the somatostatin analogue SMS 201-995 (Sandostatin) on mouth-to-caecum transit time and absorption of fat and carbohydrates in normal man. *Clin Sci* 1988; 75:345–350.

191. Moore EE, Jones TN: Benefits of immediate jejunostomy feeding after major abdominal trauma: A prospective, randomized study. *J Trauma* 1986; 26:871–881.

192. Moss G: Malabsorption associated with extreme malnutrition: Importance of replacing plasma albumin. *J Am Coll Nutr* 1982; 1:89–92.

193. Moss G: Plasma albumin and postoperative ileus. *Surg Forum* 1967; 18:333.

194. Moss G: Postoperative metabolism: The role of plasma albumin in the enteral absorption of water and electrolytes. *Pacific Med Surg* 1967; 75:355.

195. Mozzillo N, Ayala F, Federici S: Zinc deficiency in patients in long term total parenteral nutrition. *Lancet* 1982; 1:744.

196. Muggla M, et al: Postoperative enteral versus parenteral nutritional support in gastrointestinal surgery. *Surgery* 1985; 149:106–110.

197. Muhlbacher F, et al: Effects of glucocorticoids on glutamine metabolism in skeletal muscle. *Am J Physiol* 1984; 247:E75.

198. Munro HN: Free amino acid pools and their regulation, in Munro HN, Allison JB (eds): *Mammalian Protein Metabolism,* vol 4. New York, Academic Press, 1964, p 299.

199. Neptune EM: Respiration and oxidation of various substrates by ileum in vitro. *Am J Physiol* 1965; 209:329.

200. Niemiec PW, et al: Gastrointestinal disorders caused by medication and electrolyte solution osmolality during arterial nutrition. *JPEN* 1983; 7:387–389.

201. Oberg K, et al: The effects of octreotide on basal and stimulated hormone levels in patients with carcinoid syndrome. *J Clin Endocrinol Metab* 1989; 68:796–800.

202. O'Conner CR, and O'Dorisio TM: Amyloidosis, diarrhea and a somatostatin analogue. *Ann Intern Med* 1989; 110:665–666.

203. Odessy R, Goldberg AL: Oxidation of leucine by rat skeletal muscle. *Am J Physiol* 1972; 223:1376–1383.

204. Okabe S, et al: Inhibitory effect of L-glutamine on gastric irritation and back diffusion of gastric acid in response to aspirin in the rat. *Dig Dis* 1975; 20:626.

205. Olienschloger G, Sonder F: Indications and results of enteral nutrition in oncology. *J Gastroenterol* 1985; 23:6476.

206. Osei K, et al: Malignant insulinoma: Effects of a somatostatin analogue (compound SMS 201-995) on serum glucose, growth and gastroenteropancreatic hormones. *Ann Intern Med* 1985; 103:223–225.

207. Page CP, et al: Safe, cost effective postoperative nutrition: Defined formula diet via needle catheter jejunostomy. *Am J Surg* 1979; 138:939–945.

208. *Physicians' Desk Reference,* ed 44. Barnhart ER (ed). Oradell, NJ: Medical Economics Co, 1990.

209. Pomposelli JJ, et al: Longterm fish oil enriched diets attenuate the metabolic effects of endotoxin in guinea pigs (abstract No. 40). *JPEN* 1988.

210. Prasad A: Nutritional zinc today. *Nutr Today* 1981; 16:4–11.

211. Prasad AS: *Trace Elements and Iron in Human Metabolism.* New York: Plenum Publishing Corp, 1978.

212. Primrose JN, et al: Hyperkalemia in patients on enteral feeding. *JPEN J Parenter Enteral Nutr* 1981; 5:130–131.

213. Randall HT: Enteral nutrition: Tube feeding in acute and

chronic illness. *JPEN J Parenter Enteral Nutr* 1984; 8:113–136.

214. Randall HT, et al: Efficacy, feasibility, safety and cost comparison of enteral and parenteral elemental nutrition. *Contemp Surg* 1986; 28:4.

215. Rees RGP, et al: Tolerance of elemental diet administered without starter regimen. *Br Med J* [Clin Res] 1985; 290:1869–1870.

216. Reitzer LJ, Wice BM, Kendall D: Evidence that glutamine, not sugar, is the major energy source for cultured HeLa cells. *J Biol Chem* 1979; 254:2669.

217. Rene E, et al: Somatostatin and cryptosporidial diarrhea during AIDS (abstract no. 252). *Can J Physiol Pharmacol* 1986; 70(suppl):22–28.

218. Roberts WG, Fedorak RN, Chang EB: In vitro effects of long-acting somatostatin analogue SMS 201-995 on electrolyte transport by the rabbit ileum. *Gastroenterology* 1988; 94:1343–1350.

219. Robinson EN, Fuegel R: SMS 201-995, a somatostatin analogue and diarrhea in the acquired immunodeficiency syndrome (AIDS). *Ann Intern Med* 1988; 109:680–681.

220. Rombeau JL, Caldwell MD: Enteral and tube feeding, in *Clinical Nutrition,* vol I. Philadelphia: WB Saunders Co, 1984.

221. Rosen T, Mills JM: An unusual deficiency syndrome. *RN* 1981; 44:29.

222. Roth E, et al: Metabolic disorders in severe abdominal sepsis: Glutamine deficiency in skeletal muscle. *Clin Nutr* 1982; 1:25.

223. Ruderman N: Muscle amino acid metabolism and gluconeogenesis. *Annu Rev Med* 1975; 26:245.

224. Saba TM, Luzio NR: Reticuloendothelial blockage and recovery as a function of opsonic activity. *Am J Physiol* 1969; 216:197.

225. Saito H, et al: Metabolic and immune effects of dietary arginine supplementation after burn. *Arch Surg* 1987; 122:784–789.

226. Saito H, et al: The effect of route of nutrient administration on the nutritional state, catabolic hormone secretion and gut mucosal integrity following burn injury. *JPEN* 1987; 11:1–7.

227. Scheig R, Klatskin G: Hepatic metabolism of I^{14}C octanoic and I^{14}C palmitic acids. Presented at the AOCS meeting, Philadelphia, Pa, 1966.

228. Senior JR: *Medium Chain Triglycerides*. Philadelphia: University of Pennsylvania Press, 1967.

229. Shepherd JJ, et al: Regression of liver metastases in patients with gastrin-secreting tumor treated with SMS 201-995. *Lancet* 1986; 2:574.

230. Sheppard AJ, Iverson JL, Weirauch JL: Composition of selected dietary fats, oils, margarines and butter, in Kuksis A (ed): *Handbook of Lipid Research,* vol 1: Fatty acids and glycerides. New York: Plenum Publishing Corp, 1978, pp 341–379.

231. Shike M, et al: Copper metabolism and requirements in total parenteral nutrition. *Gastroenterology* 1981; 81:290–297.

232. Silk DBA: Diet formulation and choice of enteral diet. *Gut* 1986; 27:40–46.

233. Silk DBA: Enteral nutrition. *Postgrad Med J* 1984; 60:779–790.

234. Silk DBA, et al: Uses of a peptide rather than free amino acid nitrogen source in chemically defined elemental diets. *JPEN* 1980; 4:548.

235. Sketcher RD, Fern EB, James WPT: The adaptation in muscle oxidations of leucine to dietary protein and energy intake. *Br J Med [Clin Sci]* 1974; 31:333–342.

236. Skipper A: Successful enteral feeding in the critically ill patient. *Top Clin Nutr* 1986; 1:36–44.

237. Smith JL, Heymsfield SB: Enteral nutrition support: Formula preparation from modular ingredients. *JPEN* 1983; 7:280.

238. Smith PD, Janoff EN: Infectious diarrhea in human immunodeficiency virus infection. *Gastro Clin North Am* 1988; 17:587–598.

239. Sobrado J, et al: The effect of lipid emulsions on reticuloendothelial system function in the injured animal. *JPEN* 1985; 9:559.

240. Solution osmolality during enteral nutrition. *JPEN* 1983; 7:387–389.

241. Souba WW: *Glutamine Metabolism in Catabolic States: Role of the Intestinal Tract* (thesis). Harvard University

School of Public Health, Department of Nutritional Biochemistry, Boston, June 1984.

242. Souba WW: Interorgan ammonia metabolism in health and disease: A surgeon's view. *JPEN J Parenter Enteral Nutr* 1987; 11:569–579.

243. Souba WW, Wilmore DW: Gut-liver interaction during accelerated gluconeogenesis. *Arch Surg* 1985; 120:66–70.

244. Souba WW, Wilmore DW: Postoperative alteration of arteriovenous exchange of amino acids across the gastrointestinal tract. *JPEN* 1983; 94:342–350.

245. Souba WW, Scott TE, Wilmore DW: Effect of glucocorticoids on glutamine metabolism in visceral organs. *Metabolism* 1985; 34:450.

246. Souba WW, Scott TE, Wilmore DW: Intestinal consumption of intravenously administered fuels. *JPEN* 1985; 9:18.

247. Souba WW, et al: Glucocorticoids alter amino acid metabolism in visceral organs. *Surg Forum* 1983; 34:74.

248. Souba WW, et al: Glutamine metabolism by the intestinal tract. *JPEN* 1985; 9:608–617.

249. Souba WW, et al: Interorgan glutamine in the tumor-bearing rat. *J Surg Res* 1988; 44:720–726.

250. Souba WW, et al: Intestinal consumption of intravenously administered fuels. *JPEN* 1985; 9:18–21.

251. Souba WW, et al: Postoperative alterations in interorgan glutamine exchange in enterectomized dogs. *J Surg Res* 1987; 42:117–125.

252. Sox HC, et al: Clinical use of branched chain amino acids in liver disease, sepsis, trauma and burns. *Arch Surg* 1986; 121:358–366.

253. Stockmann F, et al: Long-term treatment of patients with endocrine gastrointestinal tumors with the somatostatin analogue SMS 201-995. *Scand J Gastroenterol* 1986; 21(suppl 119):230–237.

254. Tantighedhyangkul J, Hashim SA: Clinical and physiological aspects of medium chain triglycerides: Alleviation of steatorrhea in premature infants. *Bull NY Acad Med* 1971; 47:17–33.

255. Tapia R: Glutamine metabolism in brain, in Palacios R, Mora J (eds): *Glutamine: Metabolism, Enzymology and Regulation*. New York: Academic Press, 1980, p 285.

256. Taylor TT: A comparison of two methods of nasogastric tube feedings. *J Neurosurg Nurs* 1982; 14:49–55.

257. Thompson WL, Bacek LA, Powell SH, et al: Albumin versus hydroxyethyl starch in hypoalbuminemic patients (abst). *Clin Res* 1980; 28:718A.

258. Travis D, Minenna A, Frier H: Effects of medium chain triglyceride on energy metabolism and body composition in the rat. *Fed Proc* 1957; IV:561.

259. Treoloar DM, Stechmiller J: Pulmonary aspiration in tube-fed patients with artificial airways. *Heart Lung* 1984; 13:667–671.

260. Trocki O, et al: Comparison of continuous and intermittent tube feedings in burned animals. *J Br Clin Res* 1986; 7:130–137.

261. Trocki O, et al: Intact protein versus free amino acids in the nutritional support of thermally injured animals. *JPEN* 1986; 10:139–145.

262. Turkenkope IJ, Maggio CA, Greenwood MRC: Effect of high fat weaning diets containing either MCT or LCT on the development of obesity in the Zucker rat. *J Nutr* 1982; 112:1254–1263.

263. Van Buren CT: *Nutrition* 1990; 6:105–106.

264. Van Buren, et al: The importance of lymphocyte migration patterns in experimental organ transplantation. *Transplantation* 1986; 40:1–8.

265. Van Rij AM, et al: Selenium deficiency in total parenteral nutrition. *Am J Clin Nutr* 1979; 32:2076–2085.

266. Van Rij AM, et al: Selenium supplementation in total parenteral nutrition. *JPEN* 1981; 5:120–124.

267. Verschoor L, et al: On the use of a new somatostatin analogue in the treatment of hypoglycemia in patients with insulinoma. *Clin Endocrinol* 1986; 25:555–560.

268. Vestweber KH, et al: Indications and results of perioperative enteral nutrition with formula diets. *Z Gastroenterol* 1985; 23:82–92.

269. Vinik A, Moattari AR: Use of somatostatin analogue in management of carcinoid syndrome. *Dig Dis Sci* 1989; 34:14S–27S.

270. Vinik A, et al: Somatostatin analogue (SMS 201-995) in the management of gastroenteropancreatic tumors and diarrhea symptoms. *Am J Med* 1986; 81(suppl 6B):23–40.

271. Vinnars E, Bergstrom J, Furst P: Influence of the postoper-

ative state on the intracellular free amino acids in human muscle tissue. *Ann Surg* 1975; 182:665.

272. Virgilio RW, Rice CL, Smith DE, et al: Crystalloid vs colloid resuscitation. Is one better? A randomized clinical study. *Surgery* 1979; 85:129.

273. Visek WJ: Arginine needs, physiological state and usual diets: A reevaluation. *J Nutr* 1986; 116:36–46.

274. Wahren JJ, et al: Is intravenous administration of branched chain amino acids effective in the treatment of hepatic encephalopathy? A multicenter study. *Hepatology* 1983; 3:475.

275. Walike BC, Walike JW: Relative lactose intolerance: Clinical study of tube-fed patients. *JAMA* 1977; 283:949–951.

276. Weil MH, Morissette M, Michaels S, et al: Routine plasma colloid osmotic pressure measurements. *Crit Care Med* 1984; 2:229.

277. Weir JA: Trace elements in metalloenzymes. *Natl Intravenous Ther Assoc* 1981; 4:267–269.

278. Weisberg HF: Osmotic pressure of the serum proteins. *Ann Clin Lab Sci* 1978; 8:155–164.

279. Wilmore DW, et al: Altered amino acid concentrations and flux following traumatic injury, in Blackburn GL, Grant JP, Young VR (eds): *Amino Acids*. Boston: John Wright, 1983, p 387.

280. Wilson DO, et al: State of the art nutrition and chronic lung disease. *Am Rev Respir Dis* 1985; 132:1347–1365.

281. Windmueller HG: Enterohepatic aspects of glutamine metabolism, in Palacios R, Mora J (eds): *Glutamine: Metabolism, Enzymology and Regulations*. New York: Academic Press, 1980, p 235.

282. Windmueller HG: Glutamine utilization by the small intestine. *Adv Enzymol* 1982; 53:202.

283. Windmueller HG, Spaeth AE: Intestinal metabolism of glutamine and glutamate from the lumen as compared to glutamine from the blood. *Arch Biochem Biophys* 1975; 171:662.

284. Windmueller HG, Spaeth AE: Respiratory fuels and nitrogen metabolism in vivo in small intestine of fed rats. *J Biol Chem* 1980; 255:107.

285. Windmueller HG, Spaeth AE: Uptake and metabolism of plasma glutamine by the small intestine. *J Biol Chem*, 1975; 249:5070–5078.

286. Windmueller HG, Spaeth AE: Vascular perfusion of rat small intestine: Metabolic studies with isolated and in situ preparations. *Fed Proc* 1977; 36:177.

287. Wolman SL, et al: Zinc in total parenteral nutrition: Requirements and metabolic effects. *Gastroenterology* 1979; 76:458–467.

288. Wood SM, et al: Treatment of patients with pancreatic endocrine tumors using a new long-acting somatostatin analogue. Symptomatic and peptide responses. *Gut* 1985; 26:438–444.

289. Young VR: Selenium: A case for its essentiality in man. *N Engl J Med* 1981; 304:1228–1230.

290. Zagoren AJ, et al: Colloid osmotic pressure: Sensitive predictor of enteral feeding tolerance. *J Am Coll Nutr* 1984; 4:260.

291. Zielke RH, et al: Regulation of glucose and glutamine utilization by cultured human diploid fibroblasts. *J Cell Physiol* 1978; 95:41.

KEY RECOMMENDED READINGS

For a list of key recommended readings for Chapter 2, see Appendix 2, pp. 287 and 288.

SELF-ASSESSMENT QUESTIONS

Directions. Select the best response to each of the questions or statements below and then enter the corresponding letter in the space provided.

( ) 1. All of the following statements regarding enteral diets (tube feedings) are true, **except:**

    A. Inexpensive when compared with parenteral diet therapy

    B. A relatively risk-free method of nutritional therapy

    C. Preferred method of therapy for patients with a nonfunctional gut

    D. Associated with fewer technical, infectious and metabolic complications

p. 34

( ) 2. Enteral feedings are contraindicated in all of the following clinical situations, **except:**

    A. Complete mechanical bowel obstruction

    B. Ileus or intestinal hypomotility

    C. Acute pancreatitis

    D. Patients with normal gut function and protein-calorie malnutrition who had inadequate oral nutrient uptake for at least 5 days.

p. 35

( ) 3. Enteral diets are classified into two major groups, standard and special, based primarily on their protein content.

    A. True

    B. False

p. 36

( ) 4. Standard enteral diets contain intact protein, which requires normal gut function for adequate absorption.

    A. True

    B. False

p. 36

( ) 5. Special enteral diets contain protein in the form of
(low molecular weight amino acids or polypeptides,
which are readily absorbed in the presence of compromised gut function.

    A. True
    B. False

p. 36

( ) 6. The different types of enteral diets vary in their:

    A. Carbohydrate and fat composition
    B. Caloric and protein content
    C. Ratio of non-protein carbohydrate to gram ni-
trogen
    D. Osmolality
    E. All of the above

p. 42

( ) 7. Enteral diets usually contain one of the following
forms of carbohydrate, **except:**

    A. Maltodextrin
    B. Modified starch
    C. Omega-3 PUFAs
    D. Sucrose

p. 43

( ) 8. Patients with compromised gut function tolerate long-
chain triglycerides better than medium-chain triglycerides.

    A. True
    B. False

p. 44

( ) 9. Which of the following statements is **false?**

    A. MCTs are more rapidly and completely hy-
drolyzed than LCTs by the intestinal lumen.
    B. MCTs are transported primarily via the portal
vein rather than the intestinal lymphatics.
    C. MCTs are more readily oxidized than LCTs.
    D. None of the above

p. 45

( ) 10. The use of fat therapy to provide >60% of the patient's enteral daily caloric requirement may result in _____ dysfunction.

    A. Polymorphonuclear cell
    B. Macrophage
    C. Reticuloendothelial cell
    D. All of the above

p. 46

( ) 11. Most full-strength enteral diets deliver _____ kcal/cc and _____ g of protein/cc.

    A. 0.5–1.0 and .01–.02
    B. 1.0–1.5 and .02–.04
    C. 1.5–2.0 and .04–.08
    D. 2.0–3.0 and .08–.10

p. 49

( ) 12. To assure the most efficient protein-calorie assimilation, an enteral diet should have a non-protein carbohydrate calorie to gram ratio of:

    A. 100–150:1
    B. 200:1
    C. 50:1
    D. 30:1

p. 49

( ) 13. Isosmolar enteral diets (osmolality = 280 to 300 mOsm/kg of water) are routinely infused full-strength at 40 cc/hr per volumetric pump on day 1 of therapy.

    A. True
    B. False

p. 49

( ) 14. Hyperosmolar enteral diets (osmolality >300 mOsm/kg of water) are routinely infused one-quarter strength at 40 cc/hr per volumetric pump on day 1 of therapy. The concentration of the diet is then increased to full-strength over the following 72 hours before attempting to increase the rate of infusion.

    A. True
    B. False

p. 49

( ) 15. Most enteral diets contain the important minor trace metals selenium, chromium, and molybdenum.

  A. True
  B. False

  p. 50

( ) 16. All of the following statements are true regarding selenium, **except:**

  A. It is an essential component of several enzymes.
  B. It acts as an antioxidant to help prevent cell damage.
  C. It assists in the maintenance of the liver.
  D. It is present in most enteral diets.

  p. 51

( ) 17. All of the following statements regarding glutamine are true, **except:**

  A. Glutamine is the most abundant amino acid in whole blood.
  B. Glutamine and alanine transport more than half of the circulating amino acid nitrogen.
  C. Glutamine concentrations in whole blood and skeletal muscle increase markedly following injury and other catabolic diseases.
  D. Glutamine is the preferential energy substrate of the small bowel mucosa.

  p. 52

( ) 18. Since glutamine is absolved directly into the cell mitochondria and glutamic acid (glutamate) is not, glutamine fortified diets are superior.

  A. True
  B. False

  p. 54

( ) 19. Which of the following is not considered a branched-chain amino acid?

  A. Leucine
  B. Isoleucine

      C. Arginine
      D. Valine

p. 54

( ) 20. Which of the following statements is **false** regarding branched chain amino acids (BCAA)?

      A. They are rapidly consumed during periods of metabolic stress.

      B. The value of BCAA in the nutritional management of metabolically stressed patients in terms of clinical outcome is no longer controversial.

      C. Some investigators have successfully modulated the metabolic response to stress with BCAA.

      D. None of the above

p. 54

( ) 21. Most special enteral diets are routinely administered through a nasogastric feeding tube.

      A. True
      B. False

p. 65

( ) 22. Bolus and gravity enteral diet administration is safer than a continuous infusion per volumetric pump.

      A. True
      B. False

p. 65

( ) 23. The tip of the nasointestinal feeding tube should be positioned in the lumen of the small bowel (confirmed per abdominal film) prior to starting the enteral diet infusion.

      A. True
      B. False

p. 65

( ) 24. The incidence of enteral diet aspiration is significantly reduced by elevating the head of bed 30°, using a nasointestinal feeding tube, and infusing the diet continuously via volumetric pump.

    A. True
    B. False

p. 67

( ) 25. During the infusion of an enteral diet, the nurse should
check for residuals every 4 hours. If the residual is
>150 cc, discontinue the infusion for 2 hours. After
waiting 2 hours, recheck for residual. If the residual
remains >150 cc, do not restart the infusion. Instead,
contact the physician in charge for further instructions.

    A. True
    B. False

p. 67

( ) 26. All of the following are signs of enteral diet intolerance, **except:**

    A. Persistent residuals >150 cc
    B. Increasing abdominal distension
    C. Nausea, vomiting or diarrhea
    D. Improving nutritional parameters and weight
       gain

p. 67

( ) 27. Patients undergoing nasointestinal enteral diet therapy
should also receive which of the following nutritional
supplements per the feeding tube?

    A. Neutra-Phos 1 to 2 caps (250 mg/cap) dis-
       solved in 75 to 150 cc of diet four times daily
    B. Zinc sulfate 200 mg added to the diet twice
       daily
    C. Titralac, 2 tsp added to the diet twice daily
    D. All of the above

p. 67

( ) 28. During enteral diet administration, a _____ urine
glucose reading requires a STAT serum glucose determination.

    A. 1+
    B. 2+
    C. 3+
    D. 4+

p. 67

( ) 29. Hypoalbuminemia (serum albumin <2.5 g/dL) may cause which of the following:

    A. Delayed gastric emptying

    B. Decreased gut peristalsis

    C. Reduced intestinal absorption of fluids, electrolytes and nutrients

    D. All of the above

    p. 74

( ) 30. The Andrassy formula provides a method for calculating the patient's albumin deficit.

    A. True

    B. False

    p. 75

Directions. Match statements 31 to 50 with the appropriate diet or pharmacologic agent listed in A through L and enter the corresponding letter in the space provided. NOTE: The diets and pharmacologic agents may be used *more* than once.

A. Nutren 1.0	G. Amin-Aid
B. Nutren 2.0	H. Travasorb Hepatic
C. Compleat Modified Formula	I. Impact
D. Vivonex T.E.N.	J. Albumin
E. Reabilan HN	K. Hespan
F. Pulmocare	L. Glutamine

( ) 31. Preferential energy substrate for the small bowel mucosa.

    p. 54

( ) 32. Contains essential and nonessential amino acids, arginine, nucleotides, and omega-3 polyunsaturated fats.

    p. 64

( ) 33. Derives approximately 55% of its calories from fat.

    p. 62

( ) 34. Nearly 56% of the polypeptides present have a molecular weight <1,000 d.

    p. 61

( ) 35. Andrassy formula.

p. 75

( ) 36. Administered to renal failure patients (serum creatinine >2 mg/dL) with normal gut function who are not undergoing dialysis.

p. 62

( ) 37. Free amino acid, elemental diet that contains 3% fat, glutamine, the important minor trace metals (selenium, chromium, and molybdenum) and branched-chain amino acids.

p. 60

( ) 38. Intact protein, isotonic, pectin-containing diet used to treat patients with enteral diet–induced diarrhea.

p. 59

( ) 39. A synthetic plasma expander used to enhance the hypoalbuminemic patient's enteral diet tolerance.

p. 75

( ) 40. High branched-chain amino acid content and negligible amounts of sodium, potassium, phosphorus, and calcium.

p. 63

( ) 41. Intact protein, lactose-free, low-density diet for patients subjected to minimal metabolic stress with normal gut function.

p. 55

( ) 42. Administered to hepatic failure patients with normal gut function and encephalopathy.

p. 63

( ) 43. Intact protein, lactose-free, high-density enteral diet that provides 2 kcal/cc.

p. 58

( ) 44. Theoretically lowers the serum CO_2.

p. 62

( ) 45. Enhances immunocompetence.

p. 64

( ) 46. National shortage and very expensive.

p. 74

( ) 47. Contains primarily essential amino acids and negligible amounts of sodium, potassium, phosphorus, and magnesium.

p. 62

( ) 48. Provides protein as amino acids with molecular weight <500 d.

p. 60

( ) 49. Preferred diet for septic patients with normal gut function.

p. 64

( ) 50. Nutritionally more effective than glutamic acid (glutamate).

p. 52

PARENTERAL NUTRITIONAL THERAPY GUIDELINES

3

GENERAL DISCUSSION

There are two methods of parenteral nutritional therapy: total parenteral nutrition and peripheral parenteral nutrition.

Total Parenteral Nutrition Therapy

Total parenteral nutrition (TPN) therapy provides an excellent method of long-term (>10 days):

1. Supplemental nutrition for patients who are unable to consume their daily caloric, protein, and other required nutrients through oral or enteral feedings

   or

2. Total nutrition for patients with severe gut dysfunction who cannot tolerate oral or enteral feedings.

Peripheral Parenteral Nutrition Therapy

Peripheral parenteral nutrition (PPN) therapy provides an excellent method of short-term (<10 days):

1. Supplemental nutrition for patients who are unable to consume all of their daily caloric, protein, and other required nutrients through oral or enteral feedings

   or

2. Total nutrition for patients with severe gut dysfunction who cannot tolerate oral or enteral feedings.

Contraindications to Parenteral Nutrition Therapy

Parenteral nutrition therapy is contraindicated in the treatment of patients with normal gut function who are able to consume and absorb their daily caloric, protein, and other required nutrients per either oral or enteral feedings.[13, 55, 56, 59, 70, 83, 91, 154]

Parenteral vs. Enteral Nutrition Therapy

Parenteral nutrition therapy

- Is more expensive (average daily cost: $300 to $600).
- Is associated with a greater incidence of technical, metabolic, and septic complications.
- Requires more therapeutic expertise to administer than enteral nutritional therapy.

Therefore, it should only be considered when oral or enteral diets either fail or are clinically contraindicated (see Chapter 2).

Parenteral Diet Formulation

Parenteral diets are designed to provide the patient's daily caloric, protein, fluid, electrolyte, vitamin, mineral, and trace metal requirements. These diets are routinely formulated to deliver 75 to 150 non-protein carbohydrate calories (kcal) per gram of nitrogen infused. Clinical experience has clearly shown that the maintenance of this ratio maximizes carbohydrate and protein assimilation by the body, reduces the incidence of metabolical complications (aminoaciduria, hyperglycemia, and hepatic glycogenesis), and assures optimal therapeutic response.*

METHODS OF PARENTERAL NUTRITION THERAPY

The two methods of parenteral nutrition therapy—TPN and PPN—differ in terms of

1. The dextrose and amino acid (protein) content of the solution.
2. The primary caloric source (glucose vs. fat).
3. Frequency of fat administration.
4. Route of administration.
5. Infusion schedule.

*References 23, 37, 70, 91, 103, 122, 179, 216, 240, 243.

TABLE 3–1.
Comparison of Standard Total Parenteral Nutrition (TPN) and Peripheral Parenteral Nutrition (PPN) Therapies

Feature	Standard Central TPN Therapy	Standard PPN Therapy
Clinical indications	Long-term (>10 days) supplemental or total nutritional therapy	Short-term (<10 days) supplemental or total nutritional therapy
Clinical contraindications	Patients who are able to consume their daily caloric, protein and other required nutrients per either oral or enteral feedings.	Patients who are able to consume their daily caloric, protein and other required nutrients per either oral or enteral feedings.
	Patients who require short-term (<10 days) total nutritional therapy because of gut dysfunction.	Patients who require long-term (>10 days) total nutritional because of gut dysfunction.
Primary caloric source	Dextrose metabolism	Fat metabolism
Dextrose content	$D_{50}W$	$D_{20}W$
Protein content	8.5% amino acids (essential and nonessential)	10% amino acids (essential and nonessential)
Fat therapy	Fat emulsion 20% 500 cc every Monday, Wednesday, and Friday*	Fat emulsion 20% 500 cc daily†
Route of administration	Central intravenous infusion catheter with the distal tip positioned in the superior or inferior vena cava	Peripheral 18 gauge intravenous cannula or a central intravenous infusion catheter with the distal tip positioned in the superior or inferior vena cava

Infusion schedule (cc/hr/pump)	Day 1: 40 Day 2: 80 Day 3: 100–125‡	Day 1: 100–125‡
Therapeutic monitoring (CBC, blood chemistries, and 24-hr nitrogen balance determination)§	Same	Same
Therapeutic complications	Technical, infectious and metabolic (see Tables 3–6 to 3–12)	Technical, infectious and metabolic (see Tables 3–6 to 3–12)¶
Rebound hypoglycemia	Risk‖	No risk**

*Fat emulsion 20% 500 cc is administered intravenously via at least an 18-gauge peripheral intravenous or a central venous catheter positioned in the superior vena cava per pump over 4–6 hr. Fat therapy should provide at least 4%–6% of the daily caloric requirement to prevent the development of a fatty acid deficiency. The frequency and quantity of fat administered weekly may be increased depending on the patient's estimated daily caloric requirement.

†Fat emulsion therapy provides the major source of calories.

‡The final infusion rate is dependent on the patient's calculated daily caloric and protein requirements, age, and overall cardiovascular status.

§Sunday A.M.: CBC and SMAC-20; Monday (6:00 A.M.): Begin 24-hr urine collection for urinary urea nitrogen (UUN) and nitrogen balance determination; Tuesday A.M.: electrolytes, BUN, creatinine, and glucose; and Thursday A.M.: CBC, SMAC-20, copper, zinc, magnesium, transferrin, triglyceride, prealbumin, and retinol binding protein.

¶Phlebitis is the most common complication.

‖The discontinuance of central TPN therapy may result in "rebound" hypoglycemia if the patient is either NPO or has inadequate enteral caloric intake. To avoid "rebound" hypoglycemia in these patients the central TPN solution must be "tapered" or replaced with a $D_{10}W$ infusion at the previous TPN infusion rate.

**PPN therapy can be discontinued at any time without the risk of "rebound" hypoglycemia.

6. The potential technical, infectious, and metabolic complications.* The important differences between both methods of therapy are compared in Table 3–1.

STANDARD ADULT TOTAL PARENTERAL NUTRITIONAL THERAPY
General Indications

Standard TPN therapy is indicated when treating patients requiring long-term (>10 days):

1. Supplemental nutrition because they are unable to consume all of their daily caloric, protein, and other required nutrients per oral or enteral feedings

or

2. Total nutrition because they have severe gut dysfunction and are unable to tolerate either oral or enteral feedings.†

Specific Indications

Clinical settings in which standard TPN should be a part of routine care include:

1. Patients unable to absorb nutrients through the gastrointestinal tract (e.g., massive small bowel resection [>90%], diseases of the small bowel, radiation enteritis, severe diarrhea, and intractable vomiting).
2. Patients undergoing high-dose chemotherapy, radiation therapy, or bone marrow transplantation.
3. Acute pancreatitis (>3 Ranson's criteria).
4. Severe malnutrition in the presence of a nonfunctional gut.
5. Malnourished patients with acquired immune deficiency syndrome (AIDS) or AIDS-related complex (ARC) who have intractable diarrhea and no other human immunodeficiency virus (HIV)-related infection or other pathology and who are undergoing definitive chemotherapy for diarrhea (e.g., Sandostatin therapy).
6. Severely catabolic patients with or without malnutrition whose gut cannot be utilized for at least 5 days.

*References 13, 16, 21, 56, 70, 83, 91, 122, 154, 159, 203, 210, 244.
†References 13, 55, 56, 59, 70, 83, 91, 154.

Clinical settings in which standard TPN would usually be helpful include:

1. Major surgery.
2. Moderate stress.
3. Enterocutaneous fistulae (high and low).
4. Inflammatory bowel disease.
5. Hyperemesis gravidarum.
6. Moderately malnourishment in patients who require intensive medical or surgical intervention.
7. Adequate enteral nutrition cannot be established within a 4- to 5-day period of hospitalization.
8. Small bowel obstruction secondary to inflammatory adhesions.
9. Intensive cancer chemotherapy.

Clinical settings where standard TPN is of limited value include:

1. Minimal stress and trauma in a well-nourished patient whose gut may be used in less than 7 days.
2. Immediate postoperative or poststress period.
3. Proved or suspected untreatable disease state.

General Contraindications

Standard TPN therapy is contraindicated in the treatment of patients with

1. Normal gut function who are able to consume their daily caloric, protein, and other required nutrients by either oral or enteral feedings

and

2. Limited gut dysfunction who require short-term (<10 days) supplemental or total nutritional therapy.*

Specific Contraindications

The clinical settings in which standard TPN is contraindicated include the following:

1. Patients have a functional gastrointestinal tract capable of absorbing their required daily nutrients.

*References 13, 55, 56, 59, 70, 83, 91, 154.

2. The sole dependence on parenteral nutrition is anticipated to be less than 7 days.
3. Patients are in need of urgent operations. They should not have their operation delayed solely in favor of parenteral nutrition therapy.
4. Aggressive nutritional support is not desired by the patient or legal guardian and such action is in accordance with hospital policy and existing law.
5. Patient's prognosis does not warrant aggressive nutritional support.
6. The risks of parenteral therapy are judged to exceed its potential benefits.
7. Malnourished ARC/AIDS patients with intractable diarrhea who have either failed aggressive antidiarrheal (e.g., Sandostatin) and chemotherapy or have HIV-related central nervous system disease condition.

Formulation

A standard TPN solution contains $D_{50}W$, 8.5% amino acids (protein) (a combination of essential and nonessential amino acids), electrolytes, vitamins, minerals, and trace metals. A liter of standard TPN contains $D_{50}W$ 500cc and amino acids 8.5% 500 cc.

$D_{50}W$ contains 50 g of glucose per 100 cc or 250 g per 500 cc. Since the metabolism of 1 g of glucose yields approximately 4 kcal, the metabolism of 500 cc of $D_{50}W$ yields approximately 1,000 kcal. Therefore, a liter of standard TPN solution ($D_{50}W$ 500 cc + 8.5% amino acids 500 cc) provides approximately 1,000 kcal or 1 kcal/cc.

An 8.5% standard amino acid solution contains 8.5 g of protein per 100 cc or 42.5 g of protein per 500 cc. Since 1 g of nitrogen is equivalent of 6.25 g of protein, 42.5 g of protein is equivalent to 6.8 g of nitrogen. Therefore, 1 L of standard TPN solution ($D_{50}W$ 500 cc + 8.5% amino acids 500 cc) provides approximately 6.8 g of nitrogen or .0068 g of nitrogen/cc.

The ratio of non-protein carbohydrate calories (NPCC) to grams nitrogen (N_2) per liter of standard TPN solution is approximately 147:1 (1,000 kcal ÷ 6.8 g of nitrogen = 147 kcal/g nitrogen).

In addition to the hypertonic dextrose and the amino acids, a standard TPN solution contains both routine and optional additives. The basic formulation of a liter of standard TPN solution is

TABLE 3-2.

Basic Formulation of 1 L of Standard TPN Solution

COMPONENTS	
Routine additives	**Dosage**
$D_{50}W$	500 cc
8.5% amino acid*	500 cc
Sodium chloride†	0-130 mEq
Sodium phosphate‡	0-20 mM
Potassium chloride§	0-40 mEq
Magnesium sulfate¶	0-12 mEq
Ca gluconate¶,‖	4.5 or 9.0 mEq
MVI-12**	10 cc
Multitrace**	5 cc
Optional additives	**Dosage**
Sodium acetate†	0-130 mEq
Potassium acetate§	0-40 mEq
H_2 antagonist††	See footnote¶
Albumin (25%)‡‡	0-25 g
Regular insulin§§	0-40 units

ADMINISTRATION SCHEDULE

Day of therapy	Rate (cc/hr)
1	40
2	80
3	100-125¶¶

FAT EMULSION INFUSION SCHEDULE

Infuse a 20% fat emulsion 500 cc intravenously per pump over 6-8 hr at least 3 times per week via either an 18-gauge peripheral intravenous cannula or piggyback per the central venous catheter.

---

*The solution should be formulated to deliver 100-150 non-protein carbohydrate calories per gram of nitrogen infused.
†Add sodium chloride if the serum CO_2 >25 mEq/L. Add sodium acetate if the serum CO_2 ≤25 mEq/L.
‡The total phosphate dosage should not exceed 20 mM/L or 60 mM daily.
§Add KCl if the serum CO_2 >25 mEq/L. Add K acetate if the serum CO_2 ≤25 mEq/L. The potassium dosage should not exceed 40 mEq/L.
¶Added to each liter.
‖Add calcium gluconate 9 mEq to each liter if the serum calcium <8.5 mEq/L. Add 4.5 mEq if the serum calcium ≥ 8.5 mEq/L.
**Administered in only 1 L/day.
††Dosage variable. Consult the *Physicians' Desk Reference* and add an equal dose to each liter.
‡‡25% albumin 25 g is added to each liter if the serum albumin <2.5 gm% and enteral diet therapy is anticipated.
§§Total dosage should not exceed 40 units/L.
¶¶The final infusion rate is dependent on the patient's calculated daily caloric and protein requirements and overall cardiovascular status (Chapter 1).

shown in Table 3–2. Table 3–3 displays the various non-protein carbohydrate calories (NPCC) and grams protein (P) delivered over 24 hours by a standard TPN solution administered at specific hourly infusion rates.

Fat Therapy

Patients undergoing standard TPN therapy should also receive 3% to 5% of their daily caloric intake in the form of fat to prevent the development of a fatty acid deficiency.* This is accomplished by routinely administering 20% fat emulsion (2 kcal/cc), 500 cc, intravenously over 6 to 8 hours at least three times per week. Fat therapy may be used to deliver more than 5% of the patient's daily caloric requirements depending on the clinical situation (e.g., pulmonary failure).[11, 18, 87, 143, 184] It should not, however, provide more than 60% of the patient's estimated daily caloric requirement. The utilization of fat therapy to deliver more than 60% of the patient's estimated daily caloric requirement may result in the compromise of macrophage, polymorphonuclear, and reticuloendothelial cell functions.[95, 116, 136, 144, 175, 196, 223] Tables 3–2 and 3–4 show the fat emulsion infusion schedule routinely followed when administering standard TPN therapy.

Routine Orders

Standard TPN therapy orders are simple to write and should include not only the basic components in the TPN solution and fat administration schedule but also explicit post catheter insertion orders and therapeutic monitoring guidelines (see Table 3–4). Detailed, well-written TPN orders facilitate safe, efficient TPN therapy.

Adult (Age >10 Years) Catheter Selection and Insertion Techniques

A standard TPN solution is routinely administered to hospitalized, adult patients (age >10 years) via a polyvinyl or Silastic, temporary, percutaneous, 16-gauge, 8-inch single-lumen central venous catheter (SLCVC). Several of the more commonly used central venous infusion catheters are listed in Table 3–5.

Triple-lumen central venous catheters (TLCVC) are not routinely used for the administration of a TPN solution because their usage is associated with a greater incidence of catheter-related in-

*References 17, 31, 88, 120, 160, 167, 230.

TABLE 3–3.

Non-protein Carbohydrate Calories (NPCC) and Grams Protein (P) Delivered by Parenteral Diets Containing Various Combinations of Dextrose and Amino Acids*

	% Amino Acid (A.A.) Concentration								
	Parenteral Solution Infusion Rate (cc/hr)								
	6.6% AA†			8.5% AA‡			10% AA§		
Initial Dextrose Concentration	40	80	125	40	80	125	40	80	125
D₂₀W‖									
NPCC:	384	768	1,200	384	768	1,200	384	768	1,200
P:	32	64	99	40	80	124	48	96	149
D₃₀W									
NPCC:	576	1,152	1,800	576	1,152	1,800	576	1,152	1,800
P:	32	64	99	40	80	124	48	96	149
D₄₀W									
NPCC:	768	1,536	2,400	768	1,536	2,400	768	1,536	2,400
P:	32	64	99	40	80	124	48	96	149
D₅₀W¶									
NPCC:	960	1,920	3,000	960	1,920	3,000	960	1,920	3,000
P:	32	64	99	40	80	124	48	96	149
D₆₀W**									
NPCC:	1,152	2,304	3,600	1,152	2,304	3,600	1,152	2,304	3,600
P:	32	64	99	40	80	124	48	96	149
D₇₀W**									
NPCC:	1,344	2,688	4,200	1,344	2,688	4,200	1,344	2,688	4,200
P:	32	64	99	40	80	124	48	96	149

*The NPCC and P values are based upon the 24-hr infusion of a parenteral solution containing equal volumes of dextrose in water and amino acids (protein); 1 g nitrogen = 6.25 g protein, 1 g glucose yields ~4 calories.
†Amino acid (protein) concentration administered to renal failure patients who are *not undergoing routine dialysis.*
‡Amino acid (protein) concentration administered in standard central TPN and PPN.
§Amino acid (protein) concentration administered in concentrated central TPN.
‖Dextrose concentration administered in PPN.
¶Dextrose concentration administered in standard central TPN.
**Dextrose concentration administered in concentrated central TPN.

TABLE 3-4.
Standard Central TPN Therapy Orders

1. TPN Components	Recommended Dosage Ranges/L TPN	BAG No.___	BAG No.___	BAG No.___
Routine additives				
$D_{50}W$	500 cc	500 cc	500 cc	500 cc
8.5% AA	500 cc	500 cc	500 cc	500 cc
NaCl	0–140 mEq	mEq	mEq	mEq
$NaPO_4$	0–20 mM	mM	mM	mM
KCl*	0–40 mEq	mEq	mEq	mEq
$MgSO_4$	8–12 mEq	mEq	mEq	mEq
Ca gluconate	4.5 or 9 mEq	mEq	mEq	mEq
MVI-12	10 cc/day	10 cc		
Multitrace	5 cc/day	5 cc		
Optional additives				
Na acetate	0–140 mEq	mEq	mEq	mEq
K acetate	0–40 mEq	mEq	mEq	mEq
Regular insulin	0–40 units	units	units	units
H_2 antagonist†	—	—	—	—
Nurse's signature				

RATE: 40 cc/hr via pump.
Final dextrose concentration 25 % Final AA concentration 4.25 %

2. Pharmacy to add vitamin K 10 mg to 1 L of TPN q Mon. and Thurs.
3. Fat emulsion 20% 500 cc q Mon., Wed. and Fri. IVPB per pump over 6–8 hours via at least an 18-gauge peripheral IV or the subclavian catheter.
4. STAT upright and expirational portable CXR to check the position of the subclavian catheter and to R/O a pneumothorax. Notify the physician when the CXR is completed.
5. Heparin lock the TPN catheter with 2 cc of heparin (100 units/cc) until notified by the physician to start the first liter of TPN.
6. Strict I/O q shift. Total the I/O q 24 hr.
7. Record the daily weight in kg on the vital signs sheet.
8. Check the urine for sugar and acetone q shift and record on the vital signs sheet. If the urine sugar is **4+**, request a STAT serum glucose to be drawn by the physician. If the serum glucose >**160 mg%**, contact the physician for treatment orders.
9. Notify the physician if the oral temperature >**38°C.**
10. Routine TPN labs are to be drawn weekly on the days and the times specified below:

    Sun. A.M.: CBC, SMAC-20
    Tues. A.M.: Electrolytes, BUN, creatinine and glucose
    Thurs. A.M.: CBC, SMAC-20, copper, zinc, magnesium, transferrin, triglyceride, prealbumin, and retinol binding protein

11. Begin a 24-hour urine collection for urinary urea nitrogen (UUN) at 6:00 A.M. q Mon. and Thurs. for nitrogen balance determination.
12. TPN catheter dressing and tubing changes per the hospital TPN protocol.
13. Contact physician for all problems related to TPN.
14. All changes in TPN therapy must be approved by the physician.*Total potassium content per liter of TPN should not exceed 40 mEq.

†Divide the daily dosage equally into each liter of TPN.

TABLE 3–5.

Central TPN Infusion Catheters and Implantable Ports

Temporary Percutaneous	Permanent Tunnelled	Permanent Implanted
Hohn*	Hickman*	Port-A-Cath*
Centrasil	Broviac	Mediport
Pharmaseal triple lumen	Groshong	Infus-A-Port

*Recommended by the San Francisco General Hospital Nutrition Support Service.

fection.* If a TLCVC is necessary, the TPN solution should be infused through the distal port of the catheter. The clinical situations which *may* require the use of a TLCVC for TPN administration are as follows:

1. The patient has a significant coagulopathy which prevents the safe insertion of an additional SLCVC or the guidewire exchange of the pre-existing TLCVC for a SLCVC.
2. The patient has either an anatomic variant or injury which prevents the safe insertion of an additional SLCVC.
3. The patient's overall clinical status prevents the routine Trendelenburg positioning of the patient for insertion of a new, contralateral SLCVC.
4. The patient has no other peripheral or central venous access and requires continuous fluid administration, polypharmacy and TPN therapy.

A SLCVC is routinely inserted infraclavicularly into the subclavian vein, and its tip is positioned in the superior vena cava. The position of the catheter tip in the superior vena cava must be confirmed by a portable, expirational chest radiograph prior to starting the TPN infusion. The technique for inserting an adult central TPN infusion catheter is shown in Figure 3–1,A–D.[57, 59, 121, 246]

A central TPN catheter may also be inserted into (1) the superior vena cava by way of the internal jugular vein *or* (2) the inferior vena cava by way of the femoral vein. Because of the discomfort associated with a neck catheter insertion and the in-

*References 7, 47, 64, 118, 150, 155, 178, 183, 214.

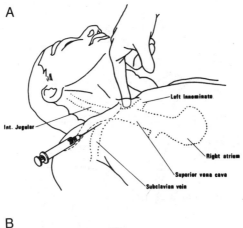

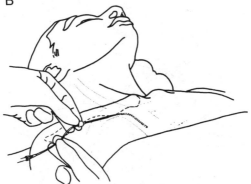

FIG 3–1.
A–D, adult single lumen central venous catheter insertion technique. (From Dudrick SJ, Copeland EM: Parenteral hyperalimentation, in Nyhus LM (ed): *Surgery Annual: 1973*. New York: Appleton-Century Crofts, 1973. Used by permission.)

(Continued.)

C

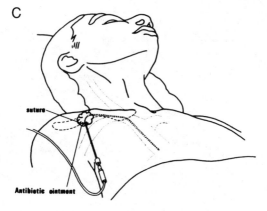

D

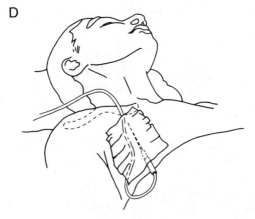

FIG 3-1 (cont.).

creased risk of infection associated with a groin catheter insertion, the author recommends the infraclavicular approach.

The TPN percutaneous catheter site may be dressed with either a sterile gauze or a transparent, occlusive, polyurethane dressing (e.g., Op-site, manufactured by Smith and Nephew United, Largo, Fla). The best sterile catheter dressing, in terms of associated catheter site infection, however, remains controversial.*

Administration of Adult TPN Therapy

TPN therapy includes the administration of the TPN solution and a 20% fat emulsion. The TPN solution is initially infused at a rate of 40 cc/hr by pump. In most clinical situations, the infusion rate is then increased according to the following schedule:

TPN Day	Rate (cc/hr per pump)
1	40
2	80
3	80–125

The final infusion rate is usually achieved by treatment Day 3. The final infusion rate is dependent on the patient's daily caloric and protein requirements, age and cardiovascular status (see Chapter 1).

TPN therapy also includes the infusion of a 20% fat emulsion. A 20% fat emulsion, 500 cc, is routinely administered intravenously over 6 to 8 hours at least three times per week. The administration of fat provides additional calories (2 kcal/cc 20% fat emulsion) and prevents the patient from developing an essential fatty acid deficiency. Patients must receive 3% to 5% of their daily calories as fat to prevent a fatty acid deficiency. Fat therapy may be used, however, to provide more than 5% of the daily caloric requirement in certain clinical situations, e.g., pulmonary failure and glucose intolerance. Fat therapy should not, however, be used to provide more than 60% of the estimated daily caloric requirement because it may compromise polymorphonuclear (PMN), macrophage, and reticuloendothelial cell function.*

*References 6, 35, 45, 114, 135, 139, 152, 161, 191, 207, 235, 241.

*References 95, 116, 136, 144, 175, 196, 223.

Taper Indications and Techniques

A patient receiving TPN therapy with inadequate or no oral caloric intake (NPO) may develop rebound hypoglycemia if the infusion is abruptly discontinued.[16, 56, 124, 238] In a nonemergent clinical situation where TPN therapy must be discontinued, the TPN infusion should be gradually "tapered" (decreased) prior to discontinuing the infusion to avoid rebound hypoglycemia. The "taper" schedule for a standard central TPN infusion is dependent on the "pre-taper" TPN infusion rate. The recommended non-emergent "taper" schedule for a patient receiving limited or no oral caloric intake with a "pre-taper" TPN infusion rate of 125 cc/hr is as follows:

- Decrease TPN infusion rate to 80 cc/hr and begin a simultaneous $D_{10}NS$ peripheral infusion at 40 cc/hr for 2 hr per pump.

then

- Decrease TPN infusion to 40 cc/hr and increase $D_{10}NS$ peripheral infusion to 80 cc/hr for 2 hr per pump.

then

- Discontinue the TPN infusion. Begin a $D_{10}NS$ infusion at 125 cc/hr by pump via the TPN catheter and simultaneously discontinue the peripheral $D_{10}NS$ infusion.

In an emergent clinical situation, where the TPN therapy must be discontinued immediately (i.e., "tapering" is impossible) the TPN infusion should be replaced with a $D_{10}NS$ infusion by pump at the previous TPN infusion rate. The $D_{10}NS$ infusion will prevent rebound hypoglycemia.

A TPN infusion may be discontinued abruptly without the fear of rebound hypoglycemia provided the patient has adequate oral caloric intake. Therefore, "tapering" or $D_{10}NS$ infusion replacement therapy is not necessary when treating TPN patients with adequate caloric intake.

Technical Complications (Including Air Embolism)

The most common complications include inability to cannulate the subclavian vein, malposition of the catheter, pneumothorax, and bleeding.*

The other technical complications that may result from the insertion of a central TPN catheter include:

- Catheter misplacement
- Pneumothorax

*References 16, 56, 63, 69, 72, 128, 173, 180.

- Tension pneumothorax
- Hemothorax
- Hydromediastinum
- Cardiac tamponade
- Brachial plexus injury
- Horner's syndrome
- Phrenic nerve paralysis
- Carotid artery injury
- Subclavian artery injury
- Subclavian hematoma
- Thrombosis, subclavian vein or superior vena cava
- Arteriovenous fistula
- Venobronchial fistula
- Innominate or subclavian vein laceration
- Catheter embolism
- Thromboembolism
- Cardiac perforation
- Endocarditis
- Thoracic duct laceration
- Air embolism

One of the most dangerous complications is an air embolism (AE).

Air Embolism

An AE is a rare and often lethal complication of subclavian vein catheterization (SVC). This catastrophic event is characterized by sudden, severe respiratory distress. In most cases, the respiratory distress is associated with both cardiac and neurologic deficits. It frequently occurs when the patient is in the upright or in a semierect position and the integrity of the subclavian venous catheter infusion system is disrupted (disconnected).

The mortality rate of the AE syndrome is nearly 43%.[180] Experiments have shown that air emboli (air bubbles) 30 to 40 mm in diameter behave like plastic beads and lodge in the smaller pulmonary vessels. In dogs, the injection of 5 to 7.5 cc/kg of air leads to gaseous accumulation in the pulmonary arterioles, arteries, right ventricle, and right atrium.[62, 131] The resultant foamy collection of blood and air obstructs the right ventricular outflow tract (pulmonary artery) and the pulmonary vasculature. This leads to significant elevations in right ventricular and pulmonary artery systolic and diastolic pressures coupled with a decrease in left heart and aortic pressures (hypotension and possible cardiac arrest). Pathologic study of experimental AE in rabbits and mice suggests that the mechanical obstruction induced by the air may be enhanced by the formation of fibrin secondary to the churning effect of the air and blood.[99, 131]

In humans, the volume of air necessary to cause significant problems is not known. It has been suggested that the injection of 20 cc/sec will be associated with symptoms and 75 to 100 cc/sec with death.[131, 173] Flanagan et al.[72] determined that approximately 100 cc of air per second could be transmitted through a 14-gauge needle with a pressure drop of 5 cm H_2O (equivalent to one deep inspiratory effort). Additional studies have shown that even smaller amounts of inspired air could be associated with significant morbidity and mortality in debilitated individuals with impaired cardiovascular systems.[62, 131]

Treatment of an AE involves proper positioning of the patient in the Durant position (lying on the left side with the head down and the feet elevated) and prompt syringe aspiration of blood and air per the subclavian catheter (Fig 3–2). The efficacy of this maneuver in cases of venous AE has been clearly reported.[41, 62, 173]

Prevention of AE after SVC relies on the integrity of the catheter system. Therefore, secure fixation of all catheter connections may prevent the complication. Peters and Armstrong[180] have

DURANT POSITION
(Left lateral decubitus)

Syringe aspiration

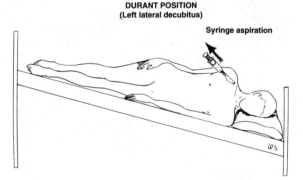

FIG 3–2.
The Durant position. (From Coppa GF, et al: Air embolism: a lethal but preventable complication of subclavian vein catheterization. *JPEN* 1981; 5:166–168. Used by permission.)

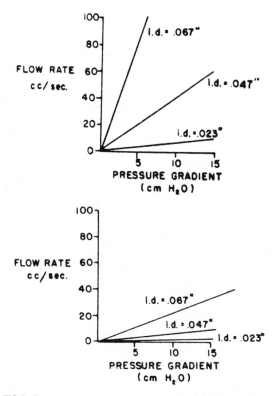

FIG 3–3.
Air flow per respiration via central TPN catheters with different internal diameters. **A**, pressure vs. flow in 5-cm tube. **B**, pressure vs. flow in 25-cm tube. (From Ordway CB: Air embolus via CVP catheter without positive pressure: Presentation of case and review. *Ann Surg* 1974; 179:479–481. Used by permission.)

clearly demonstrated that "male-female" catheter connections are very dangerous and should not be used in a subclavian venous catheter infusion system. The safest connection is the Luer-Lock (screwed together) connection.[41, 90, 131]

Ordway[173] has shown that a lethal AE can occur within sec-

TABLE 3–6.

Morbidity of Air Embolism Syndrome*

Signs/Symptoms	Incidence	No. of Patients	%
Respiratory signs	14	14	100
Neurologic symptoms	9	14	64
Cardiac signs	8	14	57

*From Coppa GF, et al: *JPEN* 1981; 5:166–168. Used by permission.

onds given adequate pre-event ventilation and the utilization of a 14-gauge subclavian catheter. Figure 3–3 displays the air flow rates that may occur with the various diameters of subclavian catheters.

Coppa et al.[41] discovered that disruption of the integrity of the subclavian venous catheter infusion system at the intravenous tubing junction was the mechanism for AE in 13 of 24 patients treated for AE. In the same study, 29% of the patients died, nearly 65% developed profound neurologic deficits, and only 50% recovered completely. Tables 3–6 through 3–8 display the morbidity associated with the AE syndrome, correlate the clinical findings and mortality rate, and serve to review the morbidity and mortality associated with previously reported cases of AE.

Infectious Complications

Patients receiving standard TPN therapy may experience infectious complications related to the central TPN catheter inser-

TABLE 3–7.

Mortality Rate Correlated to Clinical Findings*

Findings	Deaths	Patients	%
Coma	4	7	57
Apnea	3	5	60
Cardiac arrest	4	4	100
Tachypnea	0	4	0
Hypoxia	0	4	0
Cyanosis	1	1	100

*From Coppa GF, et al: *JPEN* 1981; 5:166–168. Used by permission.

TABLE 3–8.

Review of Morbidity and Mortality of Previously Reported Cases of Air Embolism*

Symptoms/Signs	Incidence	Morbidity	
		No. of Patients	%
Respiratory signs	14	14	100
Neurologic symptoms	8	14	57
Cardiac signs	10	14	72
Mortality	6	14	43

*From Coppa GF, et al. *JPEN* 1981; 5:166–168. Used by permission.

tion or the administration of the TPN solution.* Several potential TPN therapy–related infectious complications are listed in Table 3–9. Localized percutaneous catheter site and primary or secondary catheter infections, however, are the most common complications.

TABLE 3–9.

Infectious Complications Associated With Central TPN Therapy

Insertion-site contamination
  Contamination during insertion
  Contamination during routine care
Catheter contamination
  Improper technique inserting catheter
  Administration of blood via feeding catheter
  Use of catheter to measure central venous pressure
  Use of catheter to obtain blood samples
  Use of catheter to administer medications
  Contaminated solution during preparation
  Contaminated tubing via connections
  Three-way stopcocks in system
Secondary contamination
  Septicemia, bacterial or fungal
  Septic emboli
  Osteomyelitis of clavicle
  Septic arthritis
  Endocarditis

*References 3, 7, 27, 30, 47, 52, 92, 118, 119, 129, 138, 140, 150, 156, 178, 183, 206, 218, 241.

Localized Percutaneous Catheter Site Infection

A localized percutaneous catheter site infection is easily diagnosed. The catheter tract frequently exudes purulent drainage and the surrounding skin becomes erythematous and tender. If the infection is not treated, the patient may develop induration at the site. Patients with a localized percutaneous catheter site infection often develop a low-grade (38.0° to 38.5°C) "plateau" temperature, unexplained hyperglycemia (>160 mg%), and leucocytosis (>10,000 WBC/hpf). They frequently complain of generalized malaise, pain at the catheter site, or a combination of both. The successful treatment of this complication involves rapid diagnosis, catheter removal, antibiotic therapy, and reinsertion of a new catheter at a new site. The data in Table 3–10 briefly summarize the treatment of a localized percutaneous catheter site infection.

Primary Catheter Infection

A primary catheter infection is more difficult to diagnose than a local catheter site infection. Patients with this complication rarely display flagrant clinical signs of sepsis or cardiovascular collapse. Instead, the findings are less obvious. The key diagnostic triad of catheter infection (in order of occurrence) is

1. A "plateau" temperature pattern (38.0° to 38.5°C) for 12 to 24 hours.
2. Unexplained hyperglycemia (>160 mg/dL).
3. Leucocytosis (>10,000 WBC/hpf).

This triad and a blood culture positive for either bacteria or fungus aspirated both peripherally via the central catheter are highly suggestive of a catheter infection.

If a catheter infection is suspected but the blood cultures are negative, the current central infusion catheter should be removed over a guidewire and its tip sent for bacterial and fungal culture and colony count. Then, a new catheter should be inserted over the wire. If the patient's temperature defervesces and the previously aspirated blood cultures remain negative, no further therapy is necessary. A new central infusion catheter should be inserted at a new site:

1. If the patient remains febrile following guidewire catheter exchange.
2. Blood cultures aspirated prior to catheter exchange are positive.

TABLE 3–10.

Management of Infectious and Metabolic Complications Induced by TPN Therapy

Complication	Treatment
CATHETER SEPSIS	**ALGORITHMS**
Incidence	**NEGATIVE BLOOD CULTURES AND NO CARDIOVASCULAR SIGNS OF SEPSIS:**
Single-lumen catheter: 3%–5%	1. Aspirate a blood specimen per the TPN catheter for bacterial and fungal culture and then
Triple-lumen catheter: 10%–15%	sterilely exchange the preexisting TPN catheter for a new catheter over a guidewire,
Diagnosis	submit the previous catheter tip for bacterial and fungal culture and colony count (>15 is
Unexplained hyperglycemia (>160 mg/dL)	indicative of a catheter infection) and continue the TPN infusion
Plateau temperature elevation	*then*
(>38°C) for several hours or	2. Monitor the patient's temperature closely. If the temperature defervesces, no further
days *(NOTE: An isolated spike*	therapy is necessary. If the temperature continues or later reoccurs (after defervescence),
or "picket fence" temperature	remove the catheter and insert a new TPN catheter on the contralateral side and continue
pattern is usually not indicative	the TPN infusion.
of an infected catheter)	**POSITIVE BLOOD CULTURE OR CARDIOVASCULAR SIGNS OF SEPSIS**
Leukocytosis (>10,000 WBC/hpf)	1. Remove the catheter immediately and submit the catheter tip for bacterial and fungal
Exclusion of other potential sources of infection	culture and colony count
	then
or	2. Insert a new TPN infusion catheter on the contralateral side and continue the TPN infusion
A positive bacterial or fungal blood culture aspirated per both the	*then*
TPN catheter and/or a catheter tip colony count >15 peripherally	3. Initiate appropriate antibiotic therapy

(Continued.)

TABLE 3–10 (cont.).

Complication	Treatment
or Catheter site induration, erythema or purulent drainage **HYPERGLYCEMIA** (>160 mg/dL)	**ALGORITHMS:** 1. Maintain the current TPN infusion rate and begin adding regular insulin to the TPN solution in 10-unit increments until the serum glucose is maintained at ≤160 mg/dL. *(Note: The maximum allowable insulin dosage per liter of TPN is 40 units.)* Until the hyperglycemia is controlled by adding insulin to the TPN solution, simultaneously administer intravenous regular insulin. *(Note: 1 unit of regular insulin results in approximately a 10 mg/dL decrease in the serum glucose. The maximum single I.V. dose of regular insulin should not exceed 15 units.)* If the serum glucose remains >160 mg/dL despite the addition of a total of 40 units of regular insulin per liter of TPN and intravenous regular insulin therapy *then* 2. Maintain the current TPN infusion rate but begin gradually decreasing the final dextrose concentration of the TPN solution. *(Note: The lower limit for the final dextrose concentration is 15%.)* In addition, begin adding regular insulin to the TPN solution in 10-unit increments until the serum glucose is maintained at ≤160 mg/dL or the maximum allowable insulin dosage (40 units) is reached. Regular insulin should also be simultaneously administered intravenously as in algorithm 1 until the hyperglycemia is controlled by adding insulin to the TPN solution. If the serum glucose remains >**160 mg/dL** despite the addition of 40 units regular insulin per liter of TPN solution

3. Restart the original TPN solution (see **No.1**) but begin decreasing the TPN infusion rate. Also begin insulin therapy as discussed in **No.2** while simultaneously increasing the frequency of fat emulsion therapy from every Mon., Wed., and Fri. to either qod or daily to provide adequate caloric intake.

HYPOGLYCEMIA
(<70 mg/dL)

May occur with the sudden discontinuance of central TPN infusion. If the TPN infusion administered to either an NPO patient or a patient consuming inadequate oral calories is suddenly discontinued, immediately begin an infusion of $D_{10}NS$ at the previous TPN infusion rate per either the TPN catheter or a peripheral IV to prevent **"rebound"** hypoglycemia.

HYPERNATREMIA
(>145 mEq/L)

Determine the cause of the hypernatremia. Hypernatremia 2° dehydration is treated by administering additional "free water" and providing only the daily maintenance sodium requirements (90–150 mEq) per the TPN infusion. Hypernatremia 2° increased sodium intake is treated by reducing or deleting sodium from the TPN solution until the serum sodium ≤145 **mEq/L**.

HYPONATREMIA
(<135 mEq/L)

Determine the cause of the hyponatremia. Hyponatremia 2° dilution is treated by fluid restriction and providing only the daily maintenance sodium requirements (90–150 mEq) per the TPN solution until the serum sodium ≥135 **mEq/L**. Hyponatremia 2° to inadequate sodium intake is treated by increasing the sodium content of the TPN solution until the serum sodium ≥135 **mEq/L**. (**Note: The maximum sodium content per liter of TPN should not exceed 154 mEq.**)

HYPERKALEMIA
(>5 mEq/L)

Immediately discontinue the current TPN infusion containing potassium and begin an infusion of $D_{10}NS$ at the previous TPN infusion rate. Then reorder a new TPN solution without potassium and continue to delete potassium from the TPN solution until the serum potassium ≤5 **mEq/L**.

HYPOKALEMIA
(<3.5 mEq/L)

A TPN solution should not be utilized for the primary treatment of hypokalemia. The potassium content per liter of TPN solution should not exceed 40 mEq. If additional potassium is necessary, it should be administered via another route (e.g., IV interrupts).

(Continued.)

TABLE 3–10 (cont.).
Management of Infectious and Metabolic Complications Induced by TPN Therapy

Complication	Treatment
HYPERPHOSPHATEMIA (>4.5 mg/dL)	Immediately discontinue the present phosphate containing TPN infusion and begin an infusion of $D_{10}NS$ at the previous TPN infusion rate. Then reorder a new TPN solution without phosphate and continue to delete phosphate from the TPN solution until the serum phosphate ≤4.5 mg/dL.
HYPOPHOSPHATEMIA (<2.5 mg/dL)	Increase the phosphate content of the TPN solution to a maximum of 20 mM/L. *(Note: The total daily phosphate dosage should not exceed 60 mM.)*
HYPERMAGNESEMIA (>2.7 mg/dL)	Immediately discontinue the present magnesium-containing TPN infusion and begin an infusion of $D_{10}NS$ at the previous TPN infusion rate. Then reorder a new TPN solution without magnesium and continue to delete magnesium from the TPN solution until the serum magnesium ≤2.7 mg/dL.
HYPOMAGNESEMIA (<1.6 mg/dL)	Increase the magnesium content of the TPN solution to a maximum of 12 mEq/L. *(Note: The total daily dosage of magnesium should not exceed 36 mEq.)*
HYPERCALCEMIA (>10.5 mg/dL)	Immediately discontinue the present calcium-containing TPN infusion and begin an infusion of $D_{10}NS$ at the previous TPN infusion rate. Then reorder a new TPN solution without calcium and continue to delete calcium from the TPN solution until the serum calcium ≤10.5 mg/dL.
HYPOCALCEMIA (<8.5 mg/dL)	Increase the calcium content of the TPN solution to a maximum of 9 mEq/L. *(Note: The total daily calcium dosage should not exceed 27 mEq.)*
HIGH SERUM ZINC (>150 μg/dL)	Discontinue the trace metal supplement **(Multitrace 5 cc)** in the TPN solution until the serum zinc ≤150 μg/dL.
LOW SERUM ZINC (<55 μg/dL)	Add elemental zinc 2–5 mg daily to 1 L of TPN only until the serum zinc ≥55 μg/dL. *(Note: The elemental zinc is added in addition to the daily Multitrace 5 cc.)*

HIGH SERUM COPPER
(>140 µg/dL)

Discontinue the trace metal supplement (**Multitrace 5 cc**) in the TPN solution until the serum copper ≤**140 µg/dL.**

LOW SERUM COPPER
(<70 µg/dL)

Add elemental copper 2–5 mg daily to 1 L of TPN only until the serum copper ≥**70 µg/dL.** (*Note: The elemental copper is added in addition to the daily Multitrace 5 cc.*)

HYPERCHLOREMIC METABOLIC ACIDOSIS
(CO_2 <22 mM/L and Cl > 110 mEq/L)

Reduce the chloride intake by administering the Na and K in the acetate form as either Na acetate and/or K acetate until the acidosis resolves (**serum CO_2 ≥22 mM/L**) and the serum chloride level returns to normal (<**110 mEq/L**).

3. The catheter tip culture has greater than a 15 colony count.

The administration of TPN per a SLCVC is associated with less than a 7% incidence of catheter infection. In contrast, the infusion of TPN per the distal port of a TLCVC is associated with more than a 10% to 10% incidence of catheter infection.* In view of this, the author recommends the use of a SLCVC rather than a TLCVC for the infusion of a central TPN solution.

Metabolic Complications

Patients receiving a standard TPN infusion may develop metabolic complications.† Several of the more common metabolic complications and an explanation for their occurrence are discussed in Table 3–11. Tables 3–10 and 3–11 briefly discuss the management of the more common TPN therapy–induced metabolic complications.

Refeeding Syndrome

Patients suffering from severe malnutrition and weight loss (>30% of their usual weight) may develop sudden, unexpected cardiopulmonary failure following aggressive TPN therapy. This is described as the "refeeding syndrome."[101, 102, 226, 240] These patients often suffer from severe hypophosphatemia. In the semistarved or starved state, energy is primarily derived from fat metabolism which does not require phosphate-containing intermediates. The administration of central TPN results in the sudden shift from fat to glucose as the predominant fuel. When this occurs, it increases the production of the phosphorylated intermediates of glycolysis and inhibits fat metabolism. The starved patient's accentuated hypophosphatemic response to glucose is believed to reflect this shift to glycolysis and the intracellular "trapping" of phosphate.[42]

Clinical studies have shown that hypophosphatemia results in decreased ventricular stroke work, mean arterial pressure, and severe congestive cardiomyopathy.[14, 22, 50, 169] There are sufficient data to suggest that glucose induced hypophosphatemia in chronically starved animals results in deficient production of adenosine triphosphate and subsequently cellular and tissue injury.*

*References 7, 47, 64, 118, 150, 156, 178, 183, 214.

†References 8, 14, 15, 29, 42, 50, 60, 77, 84, 101, 102, 111, 117, 125–127, 137, 149, 169.

*References 12, 44, 111, 125–127, 137, 232.

Because TPN therapy can result in glucose induced hypophosphatemia, generalized cellular damage, and cardiac failure, the TPN infusion rate for a severely malnourished patient (<70% usual weight) should be cautiously increased over several days. Instead of increasing the hourly infusion rate to deliver all the patient's estimated daily caloric and protein requirements by day 3 of therapy (see Table 3–2), it should gradually be increased in 5- to 10-cc/hr increments daily provided the patient's heart rate is less than 100 beats/min. The infusion rate should not, however, be increased if the heart rate is greater than 100 beats/min.

In addition to carefully regulating the TPN infusion rate, severely malnourished patients should receive additional intravenous fat and phosphate therapy. Until the final required TPN infusion rate is achieved, fat therapy should be used to provide 20% to 30% of the patient's estimated daily caloric requirement. However, once the patient can tolerate the final TPN infusion rate, the fat therapy should be reduced to provide less than 10% of the estimated daily caloric requirement.

During the initial stages of TPN therapy, the severely malnourished patient's serum phosphate level should be frequently checked and normal levels maintained by administering supplemental intravenous phosphate. Phosphate therapy is necessary to prevent hypophosphatemic cardiac problems. Phosphate is routinely administered as sodium phosphate. The daily dosage should not exceed 60mM.

SPECIAL ADULT TPN THERAPY
Amino Acid Preparations

The different amino acid preparations available for TPN therapy differ in their amino acid composition and content. Several preparations are listed in Table 3–12 and their amino acid composition and content displayed. Because of the availability of several different preparations, nutritionists can now formulate special TPN solutions for specific clinical situations (e.g., fluid-restricted, renal failure, and hepatic failure patients).

The general indications for and contraindications to special TPN therapy are the same as those for standard TPN therapy. The route of administration, tapering schedule and the complications (technical, infectious, and metabolic) associated with special TPN therapy are essentially the same as those associated with standard central TPN therapy. The formulation of a special TPN solution

TABLE 3–11.
Metabolic Complications of Central TPN Therapy

Complication	Explanation
GLUCOSE METABOLISM	
Hyperglycemia, glycosuria, osmotic diuresis, nonketotic hyperosmolar dehydration, and coma	Excessive total dose or rate of dextrose infusion, inadequate endogenous insulin, glucocorticosteroids, or sepsis
Ketoacidosis or diabetes mellitus	Inadequate endogenous insulin response or inadequate exogenous insulin therapy
Postinfusion, ("rebound") hypoglycemia	Persistence of endogenous insulin production secondary to prolonged stimulation of the islet cells by the high-carbohydrate infusion
AMINO ACID METABOLISM	
Hyperchloremic metabolic acidosis	Excessive chloride and monochloride content of the crystalline amino acid solution
Serum acid imbalance	Unphysiologic amino acid profile of the nutrient solution or different amino acid utilization with the various disorders
Hyperammonemia	Excessive ammonia with protein hydrolysate solution; deficiency of arginine, ornithine, aspartic acid and/or glutamic acid in the crystalline amino acid solution or primary hepatic disorders
Prerenal azotemia	Excessive total dose of protein hydrosylate or amino acid solution
CALCIUM AND PHOSPHORUS METABOLISM	
Hypophosphatemia	Inadequate phosphorus administration or redistribution of serum phosphorus into the cells and/or bone
Decreased erythrocyte 2,3-diphosphoglycerate	
Increased affinity of hemoglobin for oxygen	
Aberrations of erythrocyte intermediary metabolites	
Hypocalcemia	Inadequate calcium administration, reciprocal response to phosphorus repletion without simultaneous calcium infusion, or hypoalbuminemia
Hypercalcemia	Excessive calcium administration with or without high doses of albumin or excessive vitamin D

ESSENTIAL FATTY ACID METABOLISM

Serum deficiencies of phospholipid, linoleic and/or arachidonic acids | Inadequate essential fatty acid administration or inadequate vitamin E administration

Serum elevations of 5, 8, 11-eicosatrienoic acid

MISCELLANEOUS:

Hypokalemia	Inadequate potassium intake relative to increased requirements for protein anabolism or diuresis
Hyperkalemia	Excessive potassium administration (especially in metabolic acidosis) or renal decompensation
Hypomagnesemia	Inadequate magnesium administration relative to increased requirements for protein anabolism and glucose metabolism
Hypermagnesemia	Excessive magnesium administration or renal decompensation
Anemia	Iron deficiency, folic acid deficiency, vitamin B_{12} deficiency, copper deficiency
Bleeding	Vitamin E deficiency or excessive vitamin A administration
Elevation in SGOT, SGPT, and alkaline phosphatase	Enzyme induction secondary to amino acid imbalance, excessive glycogen and/or fat deposition in the liver
Cholestatic hepatitis	Decreased water content of the bile

TABLE 3–12.

Amino Acid Preparations

Name	g Protein/100 cc	g Protein/cc	g Nitrogen/cc
STANDARD AMINO ACID SOLUTIONS			
Aminosyn	3.50	.0350	.006
	4.25	.0425	.007
	5.00	.0500	.008
	7.00	.0700	.011
	8.50	.0850	.014
	10.00	.1000	.016
FreAmine II	10.00	.1000	.016
FreAmine III	3.00	.0300	.005
	8.50	.0850	.014
Travasol	3.50	.0350	.006
	5.50	.0550	.009
	8.50	.0850	.014
	10.00	.1000	.016
ProcalAmine	3.00	.0300	.005
Novamine	8.50	.0850	.014
	11.40	.1140	.018
	15.00	.1500	.024
STRESS/HIGH BRANCHED CHAIN AMINO ACID SOLUTIONS			
Aminosyn-HBC	7.00	.0700	.011
FreAmine-HBC	6.90	.0690	.011
BranchAmin	4.00	.0400	.006
HEPATIC FAILURE AMINO ACID SOLUTIONS*			
HepatAmine	8.00	.0800	.013
RENAL FAILURE AMINO ACID SOLUTION			
Aminess	5.20	.0520	.008
Aminosyn RF	5.20	.0520	.008
NephrAmine	5.40	.0540	.009
Renamin	6.50	.0650	.010
PEDIATRIC/NEONATAL (AGE <6 MO) AMINO ACID SOLUTIONS			
Aminosyn-PF	7.00	.0700	.011
Aminosyn-PF	10.00	.1000	.016
TrophAmine	6.00	.0600	.010

*Hepatic failure amino acid solutions are very expensive and their nutritional superiority over standard amino acid solutions is currently under investigation. At this time, hepatic failure amino acid solutions are only recommended in the treatment of hepatic failure patients **with encephalopathy.**

†Standard amino acids should be administered to patients **undergoing routine dialysis.** Renal failure amino acids are only administered to renal failure patients who are **not undergoing routine dialysis.**

and its infusion rate, however, are different and dependent on the clinical situation (see **Fluid Restricted Patients, Renal Failure Patients, and Hepatic Failure Patients**).

Fluid-Restricted Patients

Pulmonary and cardiac failure patients, the elderly, patients with closed head injuries, oliguric renal failure patients, and pediatric patients often require fluid restriction. Consequently, they must be treated with a special "concentrated" TPN solution that delivers all their daily caloric and protein requirements within a limited volume. A liter of "concentrated" TPN solution contains a combination of $D_{60}W$ or $D_{70}W$, 500 cc, and standard amino acids 10% (combination of essential and nonessential), 500 cc, plus routine and optional additives (see Table 3-2). Because a concentrated TPN solution delivers more calories and protein per cc of solution, the total volume of TPN required to provide the patient's daily caloric and protein requirements is reduced.

Table 3-3 displays the non-protein carbohydrate calories and grams protein delivered over 24 hours by a "concentrated" TPN solution administered at specific hourly infusion rates.

Renal Failure Patients

Renal failure patients (serum creatinine >2 mg%) who *cannot be dialyzed and require fluid restriction,* should be treated with a special renal failure TPN solution. Each liter of solution should contain a combination of $D_{60}W$ or $D_{70}W$, 500 cc, and a renal failure amino acid preparation (essential amino acids, only) 500 cc plus routine and optional additives (see Table 3-2), with limited amounts of sodium, potassium, magnesium, and phosphate. Currently, there are two types of renal failure amino acid preparations: (1) a combination of essential and nonessential amino acids *and* (2) essential amino acids, only. RenAmin (Clintec Nutrition Co, Deerfield, Ill) contains a combination of essential and nonessential amino acids. In contrast, NephrAmine (McGaw Laboratories, Irvine, Calif) and Aminess (Clintec Nutrition Co, Deerfield, Ill) contain only essential amino acids. At present, the best renal failure amino acid preparation remains controversial.* The author, however, recommends the administration of preparations containing only essential amino acids when treating both acute and chronic renal failure patients.[1, 68, 76, 123]

---

*References 1, 68, 76, 79, 82, 85, 100, 123, 130, 185-187, 189, 201.

In contrast, renal failure patients who are *undergoing routine dialysis and require fluid restriction* should be treated with a modified standard TPN solution that contains $D_{60}W$ or $D_{70}W$ and standard amino acids 8.5% (combination of essential and nonessential), 500 cc, plus routine and optional additives (see Table 3–2), with limited amounts of sodium, potassium, magnesium, and phosphate. Since these patients are undergoing dialysis, they do not require a special renal failure amino acid preparation.

Table 3–3 displays the non-protein carbohydrate calories and grams protein delivered over 24 hours by renal failure TPN solution administered at specific hourly infusion rates.

Hepatic Failure Patients

Hepatic failure patients *without encephalopathy* should be treated with a modified standard TPN solution. Each liter of solution should contain a combination of $D_{30}W$ or $D_{40}W$, 500 cc, and standard amino acids 8.5% (combination of essential and nonessential), 500 cc, plus routine and optional additives (see Table 3–2), with the exception of limited sodium (<40 mEq of sodium/L).

In contrast, hepatic failure patients *with encephalopathy* should be treated with a special hepatic failure TPN solution. Each liter should contain a combination of $D_{30}W$ or $D_{40}W$, 500 cc, and hepatic failure amino acid preparation (high branched chain amino acid content), 500 cc, plus routine and optional additives (see Table 3–2), with the exception of limited amounts of sodium (<40 mEq sodium/L).

At the present time, HepatAmine (McGaw Laboratories, Irvine, CA) is the only solution that has been specifically tested and approved for nutritional support in liver disease patients. An abnormal plasma amino acid pattern in patients with liver disease has been reported by several investigators.* This pattern is characterized by low concentrations of branched-chain amino acids (BCAA) and high concentrations of aromatic amino acids (AAA) and methionine. The specific amino acid composition of HepatAmine provides increased quantities of BCAAs and decreased quantities of AAAs. Also, the methionine concentration has been reduced from conventional amino acid solutions. Investigators believe that high branched chain (only) solutions are not effective in patients with hepatic encephalopathy because of the increased AAA and methionine concentrations.[71]

*References 32, 34, 71, 107, 109, 158, 194, 199.

Table 3–3 displays the non-protein carbohydrate calories and grams protein delivered over 24 hours by a hepatic failure TPN solution administered at specific hourly infusion rates.

STANDARD ADULT PERIPHERAL PARENTERAL NUTRITIONAL (PPN) THERAPY
General Indications

Standard peripheral parenteral nutrition (PPN) is clinically indicated when treating patients with compromised gut function who require short-term (<10 days) nutrition:

1. Supplemental nutrition because they are unable to consume all of their daily caloric, protein, and other required nutrients by oral or enteral feeding only.

or

2. Total nutrition because they have severe gut dysfunction and are unable to tolerate either oral or enteral feedings.[24–26, 239]

Specific Indications

Clinical settings in which standard PPN therapy is helpful include:

1. Patients with an inability to absorb nutrients through the gastrointestinal tract (e.g., massive small bowel resection, [>90%], diseases of the small bowel, radiation enteritis, severe diarrhea and intractable vomiting).
2. Patients undergoing high-dose chemotherapy, radiation therapy, or bone marrow transplantation.
3. Acute pancreatitis (>3 Ranson's criteria).
4. Mild to moderate malnutrition in the presence of a gut dysfunction.
5. Malnourished ARC/AIDS patients who have intractable diarrhea and no other HIV-related infection and who are undergoing definitive chemotherapy for diarrhea (e.g., Sandostatin therapy).
6. Mild to moderate catabolic patients with or without malnutrition whose gut cannot be utilized for at least 10 days.
7. Major surgery.
8. Moderate stress.

9. Enterocutaneous fistulae (high and low).
10. Inflammatory bowel disease.
11. Hyperemesis gravidarum.
12. Moderately malnourished patients who require intensive medical or surgical intervention.
13. Patients in whom adequate enteral nutrition therapy cannot be established within a 4- to 5-day period of hospitalization.
14. Patients who have a small bowel obstruction secondary to inflammatory adhesions.
15. Patients receiving intensive cancer chemotherapy.
16. Minimal stress and trauma in a well-nourished patient when the gut may be utilized in less than 5 days.
17. Immediate postoperative or poststress period (<72 hr).
18. Proved or suspected untreatable disease state.

General Contraindications

Standard PPN therapy is contraindicated in the treatment of patients with

1. Normal or minimal gut dysfunction who are able to consume their daily caloric, protein, and other required nutrients by either oral or enteral feedings.
2. Compromised gut function who require long-term (>10 days) supplemental or total nutritional therapy.[12]

Specific Contraindications

The clinical settings in which standard PPN is contraindicated include:

1. A functional gastrointestinal tract capable of absorbing adequate nutrients.
2. The sole dependence on parenteral nutrition is anticipated to be less than 5 days.
3. Patients are in need of urgent operations. They should not have their operation delayed solely in favor of parenteral nutrition therapy.
4. Whenever aggressive nutritional support is not desired by the patient or legal guardian and when such action is in accordance with hospital policy and existing law.
5. Patient's prognosis does not warrant aggressive nutritional support.

6. The risks of parenteral therapy are judged to exceed its potential benefits.
7. Malnourished ARC/AIDS patients with intractable diarrhea who have either failed aggressive antidiarrheal (e.g., Sandostatin) and chemotherapy or have an HIV-related central nervous system disease condition.

Formulation

A standard PPN solution contains $D_{20}W$, amino acids 10% (protein) (a combination of essential and nonessential amino acids), electrolytes, vitamins, minerals, and trace metals. A liter of standard PPN solution contains $D_{20}W$, 500 cc, and amino acids 10%, 500 cc.

$D_{20}W$ contains 20 g of glucose per 100 cc or 100 g per 500 cc. Since the metabolism of 1 g of glucose yields approximately 4 kcal, the metabolism of 500 cc $D_{20}W$ yields approximately 400 kcal. Therefore, 1 L of standard PPN ($D_{20}W$ 500 cc and amino acids 10% 500 cc) provides approximately 400 kcal, or 0.4 kcal/cc.

An amino acid 10% solution contains 10 g of protein per 100 cc or 50 g of protein per 500 cc. Since 1 g of nitrogen is equivalent to 6.25 g of protein, 50 g of protein is equivalent to 8 g of nitrogen. Therefore, 1 L of standard PPN solution ($D_{20}W$ 500 cc + amino acids 10% 500 cc) provides approximately 8 g of nitrogen or 0.008 g of nitrogen/cc.

The ratio of non-protein carbohydrate calories (NPCC) to grams nitrogen (N) of 1 L of standard PPN is approximately 50:1 (400 kcal ÷ 8 g of nitrogen = 50 kcal/g of nitrogen).

Because a liter of standard PPN contains adequate nitrogen but inadequate calories, PPN therapy routinely includes the daily intravenous infusion of fat emulsion 20% (2 kcal/cc), 500 cc. The continuous infusion of the PPN solution at 125 cc/hr and the administering 20% fat emulsion, 500 cc daily, PPN therapy can provide approximately 2200 kcal and 150 g of protein (24 g nitrogen) daily. Since the maximum caloric and protein delivery from PPN therapy is limited, it is primarily used to provide short-term (<10 days) nutritional therapy for non-fluid-restricted patients subjected to mild or moderate metabolic stress.

In addition to the dextrose and amino acids, a standard PPN solution contains both routine and optional additives. Table 3–13 lists the various PPN additives and slows the basic formulation of a standard liter of PPN solution. Table 3–3 displays the various

TABLE 3-13.

Basic Formulation of a Standard Liter of PPN Solution

COMPONENTS	
Routine additives	**Dosage**
$D_{20}W$	500 cc
Amino acid, 10%	500 cc
Sodium chloride*	0-130 mEq
Sodium phosphate†	0-20 mM
Potassium chloride‡	0-40 mEq
Magnesium sulfate§	0-12 mEq
Calcium gluceptate[R],¶	4.5 or 9.0 mEq
MVI-12[R],‖	10 cc
Multitrace[R],‖	5 cc
Optional additives	**Dosage**
Sodium acetate*	0-130 mEq
Potassium acetate‡	0-40 mEq
H_2 blocker**	
Albumin 25%††	25 g
Regular insulin‡‡	0-40 units

ADMINISTRATION SCHEDULE FOR PPN SOLUTION

Start the PPN infusion at a rate of 100-125 cc/hr§§ per pump by at least an 18-gauge peripheral intravenous cannula¶¶

ADMINISTRATION SCHEDULE FOR FAT EMULSION

Infuse fat emulsion 20% 500 cc intravenously over 6-8 hr daily through at least an 18-gauge peripheral intravenous cannula

---

*Add sodium chloride if the serum CO_2 >25 mEq/L or sodium acetate if the serum CO_2 ≤25 mEq/L.

†The total phosphate dosage should not exceed 20 mM/L or 60 mM daily.

‡Add KCl if the serum CO_2 >25 mEq/L or K acetate if the serum $CO2$ ≤25 mEq/L. The potassium dosage should not exceed 40 mEq/L.

§Added to each liter.

¶Add calcium gluceptate[R] 9 mEq to each liter if the serum calcium <8.5 mEq/L or 4.5 mEq if the serum calcium is 8.5 mEq/L

‖Administered in only 1 L/day.

**Dosage variable. Consult the *Physicians' Desk Reference* and add equal dosage to each liter.

††Albumin 25% is added to each liter if the serum albumin is <2.5 g% and enteral diet therapy is anticipated.

‡‡Total dosage should not exceed 40 units/L.

§§The final infusion rate is dependent on the patient's calculated daily caloric and protein requirements, age, and overall cardiovascular status (refer to Chapter 1).

¶¶The final infusion rate is dependent on the patient's calculated daily caloric and protein requirements (refer to Chapter 1).

non-protein carbohydrate calories and grams protein delivered over 24 hours by a standard PPN solution administered at specific hourly infusion rates.

Fat Therapy

Patients undergoing standard PPN therapy must also receive a daily infusion of 20% fat emulsion, 500 cc. Fat emulsion therapy is necessary to (1) prevent the development of a fatty acid deficiency* *and* (2) provide the major source of calories. A 20% fat emulsion provides 2 kcal/cc. Therefore, the daily administration of 500 cc provides approximately 1,000 kcal.

Fat therapy should not be used to provide more than 60% of the patient's estimated daily caloric requirement. The use of fat to deliver more than 60% of the patient's estimated daily caloric requirements may result in compromised polymorphonuclear, macrophage and reticuloendothelial cells.† Table 3–13 discusses the routine fat emulsion infusion schedule followed when administering standard PPN therapy.

Routine Orders

Standard PPN therapy orders are simple to write and should include not only the basic components of the PPN solution and the fat administration schedule, but also explicit therapeutic monitoring guidelines (Table 3–14). Detailed, well-written PPN orders facilitate safe, efficient PPN therapy.

Adult (Age >10 Years) Catheter Selection and Insertion Techniques

A PPN solution is routinely infused through an 18-gauge intravenous cannula inserted into a peripheral vein. A 16- or 18-gauge single lumen central venous catheter (SLCVC) positioned in the superior vena cava through either the subclavian vein or the internal jugular vein may also be used. A 16- or 18-gauge triple lumen central venous catheter (TLCVC) (distal port) is rarely used. The PPN catheter is routinely dressed with a transparent polyurethane film dressing (e.g., Op-Site).

Administration of PPN Therapy

A standard PPN solution provides approximately 400 kcal/L, in contrast to a standard liter of central TPN solution, which pro-

*References 17, 31, 88, 120, 160, 167, 231.

†References 95, 116, 136, 144, 175, 196, 223.

TABLE 3–14.
Routine PPN Therapy Orders

1. PPN Components	Recommended Dosage Ranges/L PPN	BAG No. _____	BAG No. _____	BAG No. _____
Routine additives				
$D_{20}W$	500 cc	500 cc	500 cc	500 cc
AA, 10%	500 cc	500 cc	500 cc	500 cc
NaCl	0–140 mEq	mEq	mEq	mEq
$NaPO_4$	0–20 mM	mM	mM	mM
KCl*	0–40 mEq	mEq	mEq	mEq
$MgSO_4$	8–12 mEq	mEq	mEq	mEq
Ca gluconate	4.5 or 9 mEq	mEq	mEq	mEq
MVI-12	10 cc/day	10 cc		
Multitrace	5 cc/day	5 cc		
Optional additives				
Na acetate	0–140 mEq	mEq	mEq	mEq
K acetate*	0–40 mEq	mEq	mEq	mEq
Regular insulin	0–40 units	units	units	units
H_2 antagonist†	—	—	—	—
25% albumin‡	25 g	g	g	g
Nurse's signature				

RATE: 100–125 cc/hr via pump.
  Final dextrose concentration __10__ % Final AA Concentration __5.0__ %

2. Pharmacy to add vitamin K 10 mg to 1 L of PPN q Mon. and Thurs.
3. Insert at least an 18-gauge peripheral IV and begin the PPN infusion at 100–125 cc/hr by pump.
4. Infuse 500 cc 20% fat emulsion daily IVPB per pump over 6–8 hr via at least an 18-gauge peripheral IV.
5. Strict I/O q shift. Total the I/O q 24 hr.
6. Record the daily weight in kg on the vital signs sheet.
7. Check the urine for sugar and acetone q shift and record on the vital signs sheet. If the urine sugar **is 4**+, request a STAT serum glucose to be drawn by the physician. If the serum glucose >**160 mg%**, contact the physician for treatment orders.
8. Notify the physician if the oral temperature >**38°C**.
9. Routine PPN labs are to be drawn weekly on the days and the times specified below:

  Sun. A.M.: CBC, SMAC-20
  Tues. A.M.: Electrolytes, BUN, creatinine and glucose
  Thurs. A.M.: CBC, SMAC-20, copper, zinc, magnesium, transferrin, triglyceride, pre-albumin, and retinol binding protein

10. Begin a 24-hour urine collection for urinary urea nitrogen (UUN) at 6:00 A.M. q Mon. and Thurs. for nitrogen balance determination.
11. PPN catheter dressing and tubing changes per the hospital IV protocol.
12. Contact the physician for all problems related to PPN.
13. All changes in PPN therapy must be approved by the physician.†Total potassium content per liter of PPN should not exceed 40 mEq.

†Divide the daily dosage equally into each liter of PPN
‡Only if the serum albumin <2.5 gm% and enteral diet therapy is anticipated.

vides nearly 1,000 kcal. Because of its low dextrose content (10% final concentration), a standard PPN solution should be continuously infused at a rate of 125 cc/hr to provide at least 1,200 kcal daily:

PPN Day#	Rate (cc/hr/pump)
1	100–125

Unfortunately, most patients require more than 1,200 kcal daily. Because the PPN solution alone fails to provide sufficient calories for most patients, PPN therapy must also include the daily intravenous infusion of 20% fat emulsion (1,000 kcal), 500 cc. The continuous infusion of PPN at 125 cc/hr combined with the daily administration of 20% fat emulsion, 500 cc, provides approximately 2,200 kcal and 150 g of protein daily. Because PPN therapy provides only marginal caloric benefit, it is primarily utilized as a short-term (<10 days) method of nutritional therapy for non-fluid-restricted patients subjected to minimal metabolic stress. It should not be administered to patients who

1. Require long-term (>10 days) nutritional therapy.
2. Are fluid restricted.
3. Are subjected to moderate or severe metabolic stress.

Taper Indications and Techniques

PPN therapy may be safely discontinued, regardless of the patient's oral caloric intake, without the risk of rebound hypoglycemia. Consequently, a PPN infusion—in contrast to a central TPN infusion—does not require "tapering."

Technical Complications

The insertion of an 18-gauge intravenous cannula results in minimal technical complications. The most common problem associated with prolonged PPN therapy is the maintenance of venous access. Because of the frequent phlebitic complications induced by the PPN infusion, the infusion catheter must often be removed and reinserted at a new site. Since most patients have limited peripheral venous access, long-term (>10 days) PPN therapy is rarely possible. Despite the attempts of several nutritionists to add fat, heparin, or steroids to the PPN solution, the incidence of PPN-induced phlebitis remains the same.[19, 67, 74, 81, 110, 147]

Peripheral parenteral nutrition may also be administered through a central venous infusion catheter. The technical complications associated with the use of a central venus catheter for the administration of PPN are the same as those for TPN. The various technical complications are listed in Tables 3–6 through 3–9.

Infectious Complications

The most common infectious complications associated with standard PPN therapy are local catheter site infection and septic phlebitis.[19, 57, 67, 74, 81, 110, 147] Fortunately, peripheral catheter–induced systemic infections are quite rare.

The infectious complications associated with the use of a central venous catheter for the administration of PPN are essentially the same as those for TPN (see Tables 3–10 and 3–11).

Metabolic Complications

The metabolic complications associated with standard PPN therapy are similar to those that occur with standard central TPN therapy.* Table 3–11 lists several of the more common metabolic complications and their management and discusses the possible explanations for the metabolic complications that occur with both TPN and PPN therapy.

"Pre-Mixed" PPN Solution (ProcalAmine)

ProcalAmine (McGaw Laboratories, Irvine, Calif) is a unique, premixed PPN solution that utilizes glycerol, a 3-carbon polyalcohol, as its primary caloric source. Studies have shown that glycerol is:

1. Gluconeogenic and inhibits gluconeogenesis from amino acids.
2. Insulinogenic to a small degree.
3. Antiketogenic.
4. Chemically compatible with amino acids.
5. Higher in caloric density than glucose.

In view of these physiologic and biochemical properties, glycerol can be incorporated with amino acids and electrolytes into a single-volume, intravenous solution for postoperative protein-sparing therapy. Furthermore, glycerol can serve as an energy substrate

*References 8, 14, 15, 29, 42, 50, 60, 71, 84, 101, 102, 111, 117, 125–127, 137, 149, 169.

for patients who cannot utilize glucose due to specific disease states.†

A liter of ProcalAmine provides:

- Glycerol, 30 g
- Amino acids (protein), 29 g
- Electrolytes (sodium, 35 mEq, potassium, 24 mEq, and chloride, 41 mEq)
- Minerals (calcium, 3 mEq, and phosphate, 3.5 mM)
- Magnesium, 5 mEq
- Acetate (inorganic salts, 23 mEq, acetic acid, 9 mEq, and lysine acetate, 15 mEq)

One liter of ProcalAmine provides 245 kcal and 4.6 g of nitrogen.

ProcalAmine, although not as nutritionally beneficial as a "mixed" PPN solution, provides an economical, convenient method of maintenance nutritional therapy. It may be utilized as (1) an alternative to dextrose or saline intravenous therapy *or* (2) a supplement to inadequate oral or enteral diet therapy for patients with gut dysfunction. Because ProcalAmine is pre-mixed, its use significantly reduces both the physician's work (order writing) and the pharmacist's work (solution mixing). In addition, its usage virtually eliminates the problem of solution wastage that is associated with the use of an individualized, "mixed" PPN solution. Because of these benefits, ProcalAmine is an acceptable therapeutic alternative to a "mixed" PPN solution for medical facilities with limited pharmaceutical staffing, marginal expertise in parenteral diet therapy, or a restricted budget.

SPECIAL ADULT PPN THERAPY

The general indications for and contraindications to standard PPN therapy are applicable to special PPN therapy. Also, the route of administration and the general complications (technical, infectious, and metabolic) associated with special PPN therapy are the same as those associated with standard PPN therapy.

Fluid-Restricted Patients

Patients with pulmonary and cardiac failure, elderly and pediatric patients, patients with closed head injuries, and patients with oliguric renal failure require fluid restriction. Since the final dex-

†References 46, 67, 75, 94, 177, 182, 193, 211, 229, 231, 236, 242.

trose concentration of a PPN solution cannot exceed 12.5%, it is impossible to formulate a "concentrated" PPN solution for these patients. Fluid-restricted patients require maximum caloric and protein delivery in limited fluid volume. Unfortunately, PPN therapy requires the daily intravenous administration of 3,500 cc (PPN 3,000 cc + 20% fat emulsion, 500 cc) to provide at least 2,200 kcal and 24 g of nitrogen. Because PPN therapy requires significant fluid administration, it is contraindicated when treating fluid restricted patients.

Renal Failure Patients

Nonoliguric renal failure patients (serum creatinine >2 mg%) who *can tolerate the administration of 3,500 cc of fluid daily and cannot undergo dialysis* may be treated with a special renal failure PPN solution and daily fat therapy. One liter of solution should contain a combination of $D_{20}W$, 500 cc, and a renal failure amino acid preparation 500-cc (see **Renal Failure Patients,** p. 143), plus routine and optional additives (see Table 3–13), with the exception of limited sodium, potassium, magnesium, and phosphate.

In contrast, nonoliguric renal failure patients who *can tolerate the administration of 3,500 cc of fluid daily and who are undergoing dialysis* may be treated with a modified standard PPN solution (see Table 3–13), with the exception of limited amounts of sodium, potassium, magnesium, and phosphate.

Hepatic Failure Patients

Hepatic failure patients *with encephalopathy who can tolerate 3,500 cc of fluid daily* may be treated with a special hepatic failure PPN. One liter of solution should contain a combination of $D_{30}W$ or $D_{40}W$, 500 cc, and a hepatic failure amino acid preparation 500 cc, (see **Hepatic Failure Patients** under **Special Adult Central TPN Therapy**), plus routine and optional additives (see Table 3–13), with the exception of limited amounts of sodium (<40 mEq of sodium/L).

In contrast, hepatic failure patients *without encephalopathy who can tolerate 3,500 cc of fluid daily* may be treated with modified standard PPN therapy. One liter of solution should contain a combination of $D_{20}W$, 500 cc, and standard 8.5% amino acids (a combination of essential and nonessential amino acids) 500 cc, plus routine and optional additives (see Table 3–13), with the exception of limited sodium (<40 mEq of sodium/L).

Table 3–3 displays the non-protein carbohydrate calories and grams protein delivered over 24 hours by a hepatic failure PPN solution administered at specific hourly infusion rates.

RECOMMENDED READING AND REFERENCES

1. Abel RM, et al: Improved survival from acute renal failure after treatment with intravenous L-amino acids and glucose. *N Engl J Med* 1973; 288:695–699.
2. Abernathy CM, Dickinson TC: Massive air embolism from intravenous pump: Etiology and prevention. *Am J Surg* 1979; 137:274–275.
3. Abraham V, et al: Central venous septic thrombophlebitis — the role of medical therapy. Med, 1986; 394–400.
4. American Medical Association, Department of Foods and Nutrition. Guidelines for essential trace element preparations for parenteral use. A statement of the Nutritional Advisor Group. *JPEN* 1979; 3:263–267.
5. American Medical Association, Department of Foods and Nutrition. Multivitamin preparations for parenteral use: A statement by the Nutrition Advisory Group. *JPEN* 1979; 3:258–262.
6. Anderson PT, Herlevsen P, Schaumbura H: A comparative study of "Op-site" and "Nobecutan gauze" dressings for central venous line care. *J Hosp Infect* 1986; 7:161–168.
7. Applegren KN: Triple lumen catheters: Technological advance or setback? *Am Surg* 1987; 53:113–116.
8. Askanazi J, Matthews D, Rothkopf M: Patterns of fuel utilization during parenteral nutrition. *Surg Clin North Am* 1986; 66:1091–1113.
9. Askanazi J, et al: Influence of total parenteral nutrition on fuel utilization in injury and sepsis. *Ann Surg* 1980; 191:40.
10. Askanazi J, et al: Respiratory changes induced by large glucose loads of total parenteral nutrition. *JAMA* 1980; 243:1444–1447.
11. Askanazi J, et al: Nutrition for the patient with respiratory failure: Glucose vs. fat. *Anesthesiology* 1981; 54:373–377.
12. A.S.P.E.N. Board of Directors. Guidelines for use of home total parenteral nutrition. *JPEN* 1987; 11:342–344.
13. A.S.P.E.N. Board of Directors. Guidelines for use of total parenteral nutrition in the hospitalized adult patient. *JPEN* 1986; 10:441–445.

14. Aubier M, et al: Effect of hypophosphatemia on diaphragmatic contractility in patients with acute respiratory failure. *N Engl J Med* 1985; 313:421.

15. Baker AL, Rosenberg IH: Hepatic complications of total parenteral nutrition. *Am J Med* 1987; 82:489–497.

16. Barker BC, Weaver KE, Hickey MS: Parenteral nutrition, in Katzung BC (ed): *Clinical Pharmacology*. San Mateo, Calif: Appleton and Lang, 1988, pp 339–348.

17. Barr LH, Dunn GD, Brennan MF: Essential fatty acid deficiency during total parenteral nutrition. *Ann Surg* 1981; 193:304–311.

18. Barrocas A, et al: Nutrition and the critically ill pulmonary patient. *Respir Care* 1983; 28:50–60.

19. Bass J, et al: Preventing superficial phlebitis during infusion of crystalloid solutions in surgical patients. *Can J Surg* 1985; 28:124–125.

20. Bell RG, Hazell LA, Price P: I: Influence of dietary protein restriction on immunocompetence. II: Effect on lymphoid tissue. *Clin Exp Immunol* 1976; 26:314–326.

21. Benotti PN, et al: Practical aspects and complications of total parenteral nutrition. *Crit Care Clin* 1987; 3:115–131.

22. Betro MD, Pain RW: Hypophosphatemia and hyperphosphatemia in a hospital situation. *Br Med J [Clin Sci]* 1972; 1:273–276.

23. Blackburn GL: Hyperalimentation in the critically ill patient. *Heart Lung* 1979; 8:67–70.

24. Blackburn GL, et al: Isotonic peripheral protein sparing therapy, in *Proceedings of the International Society for Parenteral Nutrition*. September 1972.

25. Blackburn GL, et al: Peripheral intravenous feedings with isotonic amino acid solutions. *Am J Surg* 1973; 125:447–454.

26. Blackburn GL, et al: Substrate profiles in protein-losing states, in Brown H (ed): *Protein Metabolism*. Springfield, Ill: Charles C Thomas, 1973.

27. Bozetti F, et al: Prevention and treatment of central venous catheter sepsis by exchange via a guidewire: A prospective controlled trial. *Ann Surg* 1983; 198:48–52.

28. Brennan MF: Trace metal deficiency and replacement during total parenteral nutrition. Surgical Metabolism Section, Surgery Branch, National Cancer Institute, Bethesda, Md, in press.

29. Brimioulle S, et al: Hydrochloric acid infusion for treat-

ment of metabolic alkalosis: Effects on acid-base balance and oxygenation. *Crit Care Med* 1985; 13:378.

30. Brisman B, et al: Reduction of catheter-associated thrombosis in parenteral nutrition by intravenous therapy. *Arch Surg* 1982; 117:1196.

31. Burr GO, et al: On the nature and role of the fatty acids essential in nutrition. *J Biol Chem* 1930; 86:587–621.

32. Cerra FB, et al: Disease-specific amino acid infusion (F080) in hepatic encephalopathy: A prospective, randomized, double-blind, controlled trial. *JPEN* 9:160–210.

33. Chandra RK: Contemporary issues in clinical nutrition, in Chandra RK (ed): *Nutrition and Immunology,* vol 11. New York: Alan R. Liss, 1988.

34. Chase RA, et al: Plasma amino acid profiles in patients with fulminant hepatic failure treated by repeated polyacrylonitrile membrane hemodialysis. *Gastroenterology* 1978; 75:1033–1040.

35. Conly JM, et al: A prospective, randomized study comparing transparent and dry gauze dressings for central venous catheters. *J Infect Dis* 1989; 159:310–319.

36. Copeland EM, Dudrick SJ: Nutritional aspects of cancer, in Hickey RC (ed): *Current Problems in Cancer,* vol 1, no. 3. Chicago: Year Book Medical Publishers, 1976, pp 3–61.

37. Copeland EM, McFadyen BV Jr, Dudrick SJ: Intravenous hyperalimentation in cancer patients. *J Surg Res* 1974; 16:241–247.

38. Copeland EM, McFadyen BV Jr, Dudrick SJ; Effect of intravenous hyperalimentation on established delayed hypersensitivity in the cancer patient. *Ann Surg* 1976; 184:60–64.

39. Copeland EM, et al: Effects of protein nutrition on cell-mediated immunity. *Surg Forum* 1976; 27:340–342.

40. Copeland EM, et al: Intravenous hyperalimentation in inflammatory bowel disease, pancreatitis and cancer. *Ann Surg* 1980; 12:83–101.

41. Coppa GF, et al: Air embolism: A lethal but preventable complication of subclavian vein catheterization. *JPEN* 1981; 5:166–168.

42. Corredor DG, et al: Enhanced post-glucose hypophosphatemia during starvation therapy on obesity. *Metabolism* 1969; 18:754–763.

43. Cosimi AB, et al: Cellular immune competence of breast cancer patients receiving radiotherapy. *Arch Surg* 1983; 107:531–535.

44. Craddock PR, et al: Acquired phagocyte dysfunction: A complication of the hypophosphatemia of parenteral hyperalimentation. *N Engl J Med* 1974; 290:1403–1407.

45. Craven DE, et al: A randomized study comparing a transparent polyurethane dressing to a dry gauze dressing for peripheral intravenous catheter sites. *Infect Control* 1985; 6:361–366.

46. Cryer A, Bartley W: Studies on the adaptation of rates to a diet high in glycerol. *Int J Biochem* 1973; 4:293–308.

47. Crocker KS, et al: The triple lumen central venous catheter. *Nutr Clin Pract* 1986; 90–96.

48. Daily J, Vars H, Dudrick SJ: Effects of protein depletion on strength of colonic anastomosis. *Surg Gynecol Obstet* 1976; 143:593–596.

49. Daily JM, et al: Parenteral nutrition in esophageal cancer patients. *Ann Surg* Vol. 196, 1981, pp. 203–208.

50. Darsee JR, Nutter DO: Reversible severe congestive cardiomyopathy in three cases of hypophosphatemia. *Arch Intern Med* 1978; 89:867–870.

51. Dempsey DT, et al: Treatment effects of parenteral vitamins in total parenteral nutrition patients. *JPEN* 1987; 11:229–237.

52. Dillon JD, et al: Septicemia and total parenteral nutrition: Distinguishing catheter-related from other septic episodes. *JAMA* 1973; 223:1341–1344.

53. Dindogru V, et al: Total parenteral nutrition in cancer patients. *JPEN J Parenter Enteral Nutr* 1981; 5:243–245.

54. Dudrick SJ, Copeland EM: Nutritional support of the cancer patient, in Miller TA, Dudrick SJ (eds): *The Management of Difficult Surgical Problems*. Austin, Texas, University of Texas Press, 1981, pp 93–122.

55. Dudrick SJ, Jackson D: The short bowel syndrome and total parenteral nutrition. *Heart Lung* 1983; 12:195–201.

56. Dudrick SJ, Long JM III: Applications and hazards of intravenous hyperalimentation. *Ann Rev Med* 1977; 28:517–528.

57. Dudrick SJ, O'Connell JJ: Central venous lines: Inserting them safely and minimizing complications. *Contemp Gynecol Obstet* 1983; 95–103.

58. Dudrick SJ, et al: Long-term total parenteral nutrition with growth, development and positive nitrogen balance. *Surgery* 1968; 64:134–142.

59. Dudrick SJ, et al: Parenteral hyperalimentation, in Nyhus LM (ed): *Surgery Annual 1973*. New York: Appleton-Century-Crofts, 1973.

60. Dudrick SJ, et al: Parenteral hyperalimentation: Metabolic problems and solutions. *Ann Surg* 1972; 176:259.

61. Dudrick SJ, et al: 100 patient years of ambulatory home total parenteral nutrition. *Ann Surg* 1984; 199:770–781.

62. Durant TM, Oppenheimer MJ: Embolism caused by air and other gases. *Heart Bull* 1963; 12:66–70.

63. Eichelberger MP, et al: Percutaneous subclavian venous catheters in neonates and children. *J Pediatr Surg* 1981; 16:547–553.

64. Eisenhower ED, et al: Prospective evaluation of central venous pressure (CVP) catheters in a large city-county hospital. *Ann Surg* 1982; 196:560–564.

65. Elwyn DH, et al: Nutritional aspects of body water dislocations in postoperative and depleted patients. *Ann Surg* 1975; 183:76–85.

66. Fabri PJ, et al: Incidence and prevention of thrombosis of the subclavian vein during total parenteral nutrition. *Surg Gynecol Obstet* 1982; 155:238.

67. Fairfull-Smith RJ, et al: Use of glycerol in peripheral parenteral nutrition. *Surgery* 1982; 91:728–732.

68. Feinstein EI, et al: Clinical and metabolic responses to parenteral nutrition in acute renal failure: A controlled double-blind study. *Medicine* 1981; 60:124–137.

69. Filston HC, Grant JP: A safer system for percutaneous subclavian venous catheterization in newborn infants. *J Pediatr Surg* 1979; 14:564–570.

70. Fischer JE: *Surgical Nutrition*. Boston: Little, Brown & Co, 1983, pp 694–697.

71. Fischer JE, et al: Plasma amino acids in patients with encephalopathy: Effects of amino acid infusions. *Am J Surg* 1974; 127:40–47.

72. Flanagan JP, et al: Air embolism: A lethal complication of subclavian venipuncture. *N Engl J Med* 1969; 281:488–489.

73. Fleming CR, et al: Home parenteral nutrition as primary therapy in patients with extensive Crohn's disease of the

small bowel and malnutrition. *Gastroenterology* 1977; 73:1077–1081.

74. Flores-Vega CH, et al: Thrombophlebitis: Incidence using standard venous buffered intravenous solution. *Miss Med* 1970; 67:305–309.

75. Freeman JB, et al: Safety and efficacy of a new peripheral intravenously administered amino acid solution containing glycerol and electrolytes. *Surg Gynecol Obstet* 1983; 156:625–631.

76. Freund H, Atamian S, Fischer JE: Comparative study of parenteral nutrition in renal failure using essential and nonessential amino acids containing solutions. *Surg Gynecol Obstet* 1980; 151:652–656.

77. Furlan AG, et al: Acute care flexic paralysis: Association with hyperalimentation and hypophosphatemia. *Arch Neurol* 1975; 32:706–707.

78. Furst P, et al: Principles of essential amino acid therapy in uremia. *Am J Clin Nutr* 1978; 31:1744–1755.

79. Furst P, Alvestrand A, Bergstrom J: Effects of nutrition and catabolic stress on intracellular amino acid pools in uremia. *Am J Clin Nutr* 1980; 33:1387–1395.

80. Garnett ES, Barnard DL, Ford J, et al: Gross fragmentation of cardiac myofibrils after therapeutic starvation for obesity. *Lancet* 1969; 1:914–916.

81. Gazitua R, et al: Factors determining peripheral vein tolerance to amino acid infusions. *Arch Surg* 1979; 114:897–900.

82. Giacchino JL, et al: Surgery, nutritional support and survival in patients with end-stage renal disease. *Arch Surg* 1981; 116:634–640.

83. Gilder H: Parenteral nourishment of patients undergoing surgical or traumatic stress. *JPEN J Parenter Enteral Nutr* 1986; 10:88–99.

84. Giner M, Curtas S: Adverse metabolic consequences of nutritional support: Macronutrients. *Surg Clin North Am* 1978; 66:1025–1047.

85. Giordano C, De Santo NG, Pluvio M: Nitrogen balance in uremic patients on different amino acid and keto acid formulations—a proposed reference pattern. *Am J Clin Nutr* 1978; 31:1797–1801.

86. Gofferge H, Brand D: The effect of combined parenteral-enteral nutrition on the protein status of undernourished

elderly patients. *Infusionther Klin Ernahr* 1979; 6:180–187.

87. Goldstein S, et al: Energy expenditure in patients with chronic obstructive pulmonary disease. *Chest* 1987; 91:222–224.

88. Goodgame JT, Lowrey SF, Brennam MF: Essential fatty acid deficiency in total parenteral nutrition: Time course of development and suggestions for therapy. *Surgery* 1978; 84(2):271–277.

89. Govidon M, et al: Salivary secretion in hypoproteinemia states. *J Oral Med* 1985; 40:171–175.

90. Grace DM: Air embolism with neurologic complications: A potential hazard of ventral venous catheters. *Can J Surg* 1977; 20:51–53.

91. Grant J: *Handbook of Total Parenteral Nutrition.* Philadelphia: WB Saunders Co, 1980, pp 47–69.

92. Gregory JA, Shiller WR: Subclavian catheter changes every third day in high risk patients. *Am Surg* 1985; 51:534–536.

93. Grundmann R, Heistermann S: Postoperative albumin infusion therapy based upon colloid osmotic pressure. *Arch Surg* 1985; 120:911–915.

94. Hagen JH: The effect of insulin on concentration of plasma glycerol. *J Lipid Res* 1963; 4:46–51.

95. Hamaway KJ, et al: The effect of lipid emulsion on reticuloendothelial system function in the injured animal. *JPEN J Parenter Enteral Nutr* 1985; 9:559.

96. Hapariad J, et al: Limitation of central vein thrombosis in total parenteral nutrition by continuous infusion of low-dose heparin. *J Am Coll Nutr* 1983; 2:63.

97. Hardin TC, et al: Rapid replacement of serum albumin in patients receiving total parenteral nutrition. *Surg Gynecol Obstet* 1986; 163:359–361.

98. Harju E, Pessi T: Complications of subclavian vein catheters in patients with high enterocutaneous fistulas. *Int Care Med* 1985; 4:210–212.

99. Hartveit F, et al: The pathology of venous air embolism. *Br J Exp Pathol* 1968; 119:81–86.

100. Heidland A, Kult J: Long-term effects of essential amino acids supplementation in patients on regular dialysis treatment. *Clin Nephrol* 1975; 3:234–239.

101. Heymsfield SB, et al: Cardiac abnormalities in cachectic

patients before and during nutritional repletion. *Am Heart J* 1987; 95:584.

102. Heymsfield SB: Metabolic changes associated with refeeding. *A.S.P.E.N. Update* 1982; 4:1–2.

103. Hickey MS, Weaver KE: Parenteral nutrition, in Luce JM, Pierson DJ (eds): *Critical Care Medicine*. Philadelphia, WB Saunders Co, 1988, pp 374–378.

104. Horbst CA Jr: Indications, management and complications of percutaneous subclavian catheters. *Arch Surg* 1978; 113:1421–1425.

105. Howland WS, et al: Colloid oncotic pressure and levels of albumin and total protein during major surgical procedures *Surg Gynecol Obstet* 1976; 143:592–596.

106. Hull RL: Use of trace elements in intravenous hyperalimentation solutions. *Am J Hosp Pharm* 1974; 31:759.

107. Iber FL, et al: The plasma amino acids in patients with liver failure. *J Lab Clin Med* 1957; 50:417–425.

108. Inculet RI, et al: Water-soluble vitamins in cancer patients on parenteral nutrition: A prospective study. *JPEN* 1987; 11:248–249.

109. Iob V, Coon W, Sloan M: Altered clearance of free amino acids from patients with cirrhosis of the liver. *J Surg Res* 1966; 6:233.

110. Isaacs JW, et al: Parenteral nutrition of adults with 900 milliosmolar solution via peripheral veins. *Am J Clin Nutr* 1977; 3:552–559.

111. Jacobs HS, Amsden T: Acute hemolytic anemia with rigid red cells in hypophosphatemia. *N Engl J Med* 1971; 285:1446–1450.

112. Jacobsen S, Kallner A: Effect of total parenteral nutrition on serum concentrations of eight proteins in Crohn's disease. *Am J Gastroenterol* 1985; 79:501–505.

113. Jarrard M: Use of transparent polyurethane dressing for central venous catheter care. Presented at the A.S.P.E.N. 4th Clinical Congress, January 1980.

114. Jarrard MM, et al: Daily dressing change effects on skin flora beneath subclavian catheter dressings during total parenteral nutrition. *JPEN* 1980; 4:391–392.

115. Jeejeebhoy KN, et al: Total parenteral nutrition at home: Studies in patients surviving 4 months to 5 years. *Gastroenterology* 1976; 71:943–953.

116. Jensen GL, et al: Parenteral infusion of medium chain tri-

glycerides and reticuloendothelial system function in man. *Am J Clin Nutr* 1988; 47:786.

117. Juan D: The causes and consequences of hypophosphatemia. *Surg Gynecol Obstet* 1982; 153:589.

118. Kaufman J, et al: Catheter-related septic central venous thrombosis—current therapeutic options. *West J Med* 1986; 145:200–203.

119. Kaufman JL, et al: Clinical experience with the multiple lumen central venous catheter. *JPEN* 1986; 10:487–489.

120. Kellenberger TA, et al: Essential fatty acid deficiency: A consequence of fat-free total parenteral nutrition. *Am J Hosp Pharm* 1979; 36:230–234.

121. Kenney PR, et al: Percutaneous inferior vena cava cannulation for long-term parenteral nutrition. *Surgery* 1985; 97:602–604.

122. Kilpatrick Jr, et al: The therapeutic advantages in a balanced nutritional support system. *Ann Surg* 1981; 89:370.

123. Kjellstrand CM, Ebben J, Davin T: Time of death, recovery of renal function, development of chronic renal failure and need for chronic hemodialysis in patients with acute tubular necrosis. *Trans Am Soc Artif Intern Organs* 1981; 27:45–50.

124. Klein GL, Riva D: Adverse metabolic consequences of total parenteral nutrition. *Cancer* 1985; 55:305–308.

125. Klock JC, Williams HE, Mentzer WC: Hemolytic anemia and somatic cell dysfunction in severe hypophosphatemia. *Arch Intern Med* 1974; 134:360–364.

126. Knochel JP: The pathophysiology and clinical characteristic of severe hypophosphatemia. *Arch Intern Med* 1977; 137:203–220.

127. Knochel JP, et al: Hypophosphatemia and rhabdomyolysis. *J Clin Invest* 1978; 62:1240–1246.

128. Kobloske AM, Klein ME: Technique of central venous access for long-term parenteral nutrition in infants. *Surg Gynecol Obstet* 1982; 154:395–399.

129. Konnista K, et al: The subclavian vein catheter related infections. *Anesth Analg* 1981; 38:645–650.

130. Kopple JD: Treatment of renal failure with defined-formula diets, in *Defined Formula Diets for Medical Purposes*. Chicago: American Medical Association, 1979.

131. Lambert MJ: Air embolism in central venous catheterization: Diagnosis, treatment and prevention. *South Med J* 1982; 75:1189–1191.

132. Law DK, Dudrick SJ, Abdou NI: The effect of dietary protein depletion on immunocompetence: The importance of nutritional repletion prior to immunological induction. *Ann Surg* 1974; 179:168–173.

133. Law DK, Dudrick SJ, Abdou NI: The effects of protein-calorie malnutrition on immune competence of the surgical patient. *Surg Gynecol Obstet* 1974; 139:266.

134. Law DK, Dudrick SJ, Abdou NI: Immunocompetence of patients with protein-calorie malnutrition: The effects of nutritional repletion. *Ann Intern Med* 1973; 79:545–550.

135. Lawson M, et al: Comparison of transport dressings to paper tape dressing over central venous catheter sites. *Nursing Intravenous Therapy Association* 1986; 9:40–43.

136. Lee TH, et al: Effect of dietary and enrichment with eicosapentaenoic acids in vitro neutrophil and monocyte leukotriene generation and neutrophil function. *N Engl J Med* 1985; 312:1217.

137. Lichtman MA, et al: Reduced red cell glycolysis 2,3-diphosphoglycerate and adenosine triphosphate concentration, and increased hemoglobin-oxygen affinity caused by hypophosphatemia. *Ann Intern Med* 1971; 74:562–568.

138. Linares J, et al: Pathogenesis of catheter sepsis: A prospective study with quantitative and semi-quantitative cultures of catheter hub and segments. *J Clin Microbiol* 1985; 21:357–360.

139. Littenberg B, Thompson L: Gauze vs. plastic for peripheral intravenous dressings: Testing a new technology. *J Gen Intern Med* 1987; 2:411–414.

140. Lodegode K, et al: I: Long-term parenteral nutrition. II: Catheter-related complications. *Scan J Gastroenterol* 1981; 16:913–919.

141. Lul H, Saini AS: Leukocyte free amino acid alteration in hypoproteinemic conditions. *Indian J Pediatr* 1986; 23:209–212.

142. Lundholm K, et al: Is it possible to evaluate the efficacy of amino acid solutions after major surgical procedures or accidental injuries? *JPEN* 1986; 10:29–33.

143. MacFadyen BV, et al: Management of gastrointestinal fistulas with parenteral hyperalimentation. *Surgery* 1973; 74:100–105.

144. Magrum, et al: Effect of culture in vitro with eicosatetraenoic and eicosapentaenoic acids in fatty acid composition, prostaglandin synthesis and chemiluminescence of rat

peritoneal macrophages. *Biochem Biophys Acta* 1984; 863:354.

145. Maix A, et al: Effect on DL-3-hydroxybutyrate infusions on leucine and glucose kinetic in burned rates receiving RPN. *J Nutr* 1986; 116:149–156.

146. Makarewicz PA, et al: Prevention of superficial phlebitis during peripheral parenteral nutrition. *Am J Surg* 1986; 151:124–129.

147. Maki DG, Weise CE, Sarafin MW: A semi-quantitative culture method for identifying intravenous catheter-related infection. *N Engl J Med* 1977; 296:1305–1309.

148. Mattar JA, et al: Parenteral nutrition as a useful method for weaning patients from mechanical ventilation (abstract 50). *JPEN* 1978; 2:26–30.

149. McAuliffe W, et al: Hypoproteinemic alkalosis. *Am J Med* 1986; 81:86–90.

150. McCarthy MC, et al: Prospective evaluation of single and triple lumen catheters in total parenteral nutrition. *JPEN* 1987; 11:259–262.

151. McCauley RL, Brennan MF: Serum albumin levels in cancer patients receiving total parenteral nutrition. *Ann Surg* 1983; 197:305.

152. McCredie KB, et al: A comparative evaluation of transparent dressings and gauze dressings for central venous catheters. *JPEN* 1984; 8:96.

153. McFie J, et al: Effect of energy source on changes in energy expenditure and respiratory quotient during total parenteral nutrition. *JPEN* 1983; 7:1–5.

154. Mequid M, et al: The delivery of nutritional support. A potpourri of new devices and methods. *Cancer* 1985; 1:279–289.

155. Michel L: Microbial colonization of indwelling central venous catheters: Statistical evaluation of potential contaminating factors. *Am J Surg* 1979; 137:745–748.

156. Miller, et al: Comparison of the sterility of long-term central venous catheterization using single lumen, triple lumen and pulmonary artery catheters. *Crit Care Med* 1984; 12:634–637.

157. Mirtallo JM, et al: Albumin in TPN Solutions: Potential savings from a prospective review. *JPEN* 1980; 4:300–302.

158. Morgan MY, Milson JP, Sherlock S: Plasma ration of va-

line, leucine and isoleucine to phenylalanine and tyrosine in liver disease. *Gut* 1978; 19:1061–1073.

159. Mullen J: Consequences of malnutrition in the surgical patient. *Surg Clin North Am* 1989; 61:169.

160. National Academy of Sciences. *Recommended Dietary Allowances,* ed 9. Washington, DC: 1980, pp 33–35.

161. Nehme AE, Trigger JA: Catheter dressings in central venous parenteral nutrition: A prospective randomized comparative study. *Nutr Suppl Serv* 1984; 4:42–50.

162. Nelane AE: Nutritional support of the hospitalized patient. The team concept. *JAMA* 1980; 246:1906–1908.

163. Newsome HH Jr, et al: Mechanical complications from insertion of subclavian venous feeding catheters: Comparison of de novo percutaneous venipuncture to change of catheter over guidewire. *JPEN* 1984; 8:560–562.

164. Nixon DW, et al: Hyperalimentation of the cancer patient with n-calorie undernutrition. *Cancer Res* 1981; 41:2038–2045.

165. Nonji AA, et al: Hyperuricemia and hypoalbuminemia predispose to cisplatin-induced nephrotoxicity. *Cancer Chemother Pharmacol* 1986; 17:274–276.

166. Nordenstrom J, et al: Nitrogen balance during total parenteral nutrition. *Ann Surg* 1983; 197:27–33.

167. Nordenstrom J, et al: Metabolic utilization of intravenous fat emulsion during total parenteral nutrition. *Ann Surg* 1982; 196:221–230.

168. Novozhilov V: Evaluation of complications of subclavian vein catheterization. *Anesteziol Renrimatol* 1982; 4:65–66.

169. O'Connor LR, Wheeler WS, Bethune JE: Effect of hypophosphatemia on myocardial performance in man. *N Engl J Med* 1977; 297:901–903.

170. O'Donnell JJ, et al: Percutaneous insertion of a cuffed catheter with a long subcutaneous tunnel for intravenous hyperalimentation. *South Med J* 1983; 76:1344–1348.

171. Ohno R, Hersch EM: Immunosuppressive effects of L-asparaginase. *Cancer Res* 1970; 30:1605–1611.

172. Oppenheimer MJ, Durant TM, Lynch P: Body position in relation to venous air embolism and the associated cardiovascular respiratory changes. *Am J Med Sci* 1953; 225:362–373.

173. Ordway CB: Air embolism via CVP catheter without positive pressure. *Ann Surg* 1974; 179:479–481.

174. Ostro MJ, et al: Total parenteral nutrition and complete bowel rest in the management of Crohn's disease. *JPEN* 1985; 9:280–287.

175. Ota DM, et al: Effects of intralipid on lymphocyte transformation. *Fed Proc* 1977; 36:1218.

176. Palidor PJ, Siminowitz DA, Oneskovich MR: Use of opsite as an occlusive dressing for total parenteral nutrition catheters. *JPEN* 1982; 6:150–151.

177. Pelkonen R, Nikkila EA, Kekki M: Metabolism of glycerol in diabetes mellitus. *Diabetologia* 1968; 3:1–8.

178. Pemberton LB, et al: Sepsis from triple vs. single-lumen catheters during total parenteral nutrition in surgical or critically ill patients. *Arch Surg* 1986; 121:591–594.

179. Peters C, Fischer JE: Studies on calorie to nitrogen ratio for total parenteral nutrition. *Surg Gynecol Obstet* 1980; 151:1–8.

180. Peters JL, Armstrong R: Air embolism occurring as a complication of central venous catheterization. *Ann Surg* 1978; 187:375–378.

181. Peters T Jr, Peters JC: The biosynthesis of rat serum albumin. *J Biol Chem* 1972; 247:3858–3863.

182. Phadke AS, et al: Intravenous glycerol in increased intracranial tension. *J Assoc Physicians India* 1975; 24:147–151.

183. Pine RW, et al: The triple lumen central venous catheter, in *Nutrition in Clinical Practice*. Silver Spring, Md: American Society for Parenteral and Enteral Nutrition, 1986.

184. Pingleton SK: Nutrition in acute respiratory failure. *Lung* 1986; 164:127–137.

185. Pitts RF: The effects of infusing glycine and of varying the dietary protein intake on renal hemodynamics in the dog. *Am J Physiol* 1944; 142:355–365.

186. Pitts RF: Metabolism of amino acids by the perfused rat kidney. *Am J Physiol* 1971; 220:862–867.

187. Pitts RF: The role of ammonia production and excretion in regulation of acid-base balance. *N Engl J Med* 1971; 284:32–38.

188. Piraino AJ, Firpo JJ, Powers DV: Prolonged hyperalimentation in catabolic chronic dialysis therapy patients. *JPEN* 1981; 5:463–477.

189. Poliakoff CB, et al: The removal of central venous silicone rubber catheters. *JAMA* 1986; 255:2021–2022.

190. Popp MB, et al: A prospective randomized study of adjuvant parenteral nutrition in the treatment of diffuse lymphoma: Effect on drug tolerance. *Cancer Treat Rep* 1981; 65:129–135.

191. Powell C, et al: Evaluation of op-site catheter dressings for parenteral nutrition: A prospective, randomized study. *JPEN* 1982; 6:43–46.

192. Rapp RP, et al: The favorable effect of early parenteral feeding on survival in head-injured patients. *J Neurosurg* 1983; 58:906–912.

193. Reinglass JL: Dose response curve to intravenous glycerol in the treatment of cerebral edema due to trauma. *Neurology* 1974; 24:743–747.

194. Richmond J, Girdwood R: Observations on amino acid absorption. *Clin Sci* 1962; 22:301.

195. Riggle MA, Brandt RB: Decrease of available vitamin A in parenteral nutrition solutions. *JPEN* 1986; 10:388–391.

196. Ring, et al: Prolongation of skin allografts in rats by treatment with linoleic acid. *Lancet* 1974; 2:1331–1333.

197. Ringsdorf WM, et al: Vitamin C and human wound healing. *Oral Surg* 1982; 53:231–236.

198. Rombeau JL, Caldwell MD: *Clinical Nutrition,* vol II. *Parenteral Nutrition.* Philadelphia: WB Saunders Co, 1986.

199. Rosen HM, et al: Plasma amino acid patterns in hepatic encephalopathy of differing etiology. *Gastroenterology* 1977; 72:483–487.

200. Rowlands BJ, et al: Selenium depletion in burn patients. *JPEN* 1984; 8:365.

201. Rudman D, et al: Comparison of the effect of various amino acids upon the blood ammonia concentration of patients with liver disease. *Am J Clin Nutr* 1973; 26:916–925.

202. Rutten P, et al: Determination of optimal hyperalimentation infusion rate. *J Surg Res* 1975; 18:477–483.

203. Ryan JA, et al: Catheter complication in total parenteral nutrition: A prospective study of 200 consecutive patients. *N Engl J Med* 1974; 290:757–761.

204. Ryzen E, et al: Magnesium deficiency in a medical ICU population. *Crit Care Med* 1985; 13:19.

205. Sakamoto J, et al: The effect of intravenous hyperalimentation on cell mediated immunity. *J Surg* 1979; 9:89–94.

206. Saunders JE, et al: Experience with double lumen right atrial catheters. *JPEN* 1982; 6:95–99.

207. Schwartz-Fulton J, et al: Hyperalimentation dressing and skin flora. *Nursing Intravenous Therapy Association* 1981; 4:354–357.

208. Schwartz S, et al: Evaluation of protein metabolism and albumin in patients submitted to peripheral parenteral nutrition (PPN). *Infusionsther Klin Ernahr* 1984; 11:137–140.

209. Seifer DB, et al: Total parenteral nutrition in obstetrics. *JAMA* 1985; 253:2073–2075.

210. Seifort W: Metabolic problems of malnutrition in cancer patients and the treatment of parenteral substitution. *Arch Geschwulstforsch* 1981; 51:434–441.

211. Seniro B, Loridan L: Studies of liver glycogenesis with particular reference to the metabolism of intravenously administered glycerol. *N Engl J Med* 1968; 279:958–965.

212. Sheldon GF: Septic complications of total parenteral nutrition. *Surgery* 1976; 132:214–218.

213. Shenkin A: Vitamin and essential element recommendations during intravenous nutrition: Therapy and practice. *Proc Nutr Soc* 1986; 45:383–390.

214. Sherman RA, et al: Multilumen catheter sepsis and an educational process to combat it. *Am J Infect Control* 1988; 16:31A–34A.

215. Shizgal HM, Forse RA: Protein and calorie requirements with total parenteral nutrition. *Ann Surg* 1980; 192:562–569.

216. Silberman H: The role of postoperative parenteral nutrition in cancer patients. *Cancer* 1985; 1:354–357.

217. Silberman H, et al: The safety and efficacy of a lipid-based system of parenteral nutrition in acute pancreatitis. *Gastroenterology* 1982; 77:494–497.

218. Sitges-Serra A, Linares J, Garau J: Catheter sepsis: The clue is the hub. *Surgery* 1985; 98:355–357.

219. Skillman W, et al: Improved albumin synthesis in postoperative patients by amino acid infusion. *N Engl J Med* 1976; 293:1037–1040.

220. Skillman W, et al: Energy intake can determine albumin synthesis in man after injury. *Surgery* 1985; 97:272–276.

221. Slade MS, et al: Immunodepression after major surgery in normal patients. *Surgery* 1975; 78:363–372.

222. Smythe PM, et al: Thymolymphatic deficiency and depres-

sion of cell-mediated immunity in protein-calorie malnutrition. *Lancet* 1971; 2:939–944.

223. Sobrado, et al: Lipid emulsion and reticuloendothelial system function in healthy and burned guinea pigs. *Am J Clin Nutr* 1986; 42:855.

224. Somsygina GA, Shilenkova VI: Syndrome of compression of the superior vena cava caused by catheterization of the subclavian vein in newborn infants with septicemia. *Pediatria* 1982; 10:60–61.

225. Soule BM: *The APIC Curriculum for Infection Control Practice*. Dubuque, Iowa: Kendall/Hunt, 1983, p 602.

226. Starker PM, et al: Response to total parenteral nutrition in the extremely malnourished patient. *JPEN* 1985; 9:300–302.

227. Storbel CT, et al: Home parenteral nutrition in children with Crohn's disease: An effective management alternative. *Gastroenterology* 1979; 77:272–279.

228. Suddleson EA: Cardiac tamponade: A complication of central venous hyperalimentation. *JPEN* 1986; 10:528–529.

229. Tac RC, et al: Glycerol: Its metabolism and use as an intravenous energy source. *JPEN* 1983; 7:479–487.

230. Tashiro T, et al: The effect of fat emulsion on essential fatty acid deficiency during intravenous hyperalimentation in pediatric patients. *J Pediatr Surg* 1975; 10:203–213.

231. Tourtellotte WW, et al: Cerebral dehydration action of glycerol. I: Historical aspects with emphasis on the toxicity and intravenous administration. *Clin Pharmacol Ther* 1972; 13:159–171.

232. Travis SF, et al: Alterations of red-cell glycolytic intermediates and oxygen transport as a consequence of hypophosphatemia in patients receiving intravenous hyperalimentation. *N Engl J Med* 1971; 285:763–768.

233. Tullis J: Albumin. II: Guidelines for clinical use. *JAMA* 1977; 237:460–463.

234. Twyman D, et al: Fat emulsions as a calorie source in total parenteral nutrition. *Am J Intra Ther Clin Nutr* 1982.

235. Vazquez RN, Jarrard MM: Care of central venous catheterization site: The use of transparent polyurethane film. *JPEN* 1980; 8:181–186.

236. Vernon RG, Walker DG: Glycerol metabolism in the neonatal rat. *Biochem J* 1970; 118:531–536.

237. Von Meyenfeldt MM, et al: TPN catheter sepsis: Lack of

effect on subcutaneous tunnelling of PVC catheters on sepsis rate. *JPEN* 1980; 4:514–517.

238. Wagman LD, et al: The effect of acute discontinuation of total parenteral nutrition. *Ann Surg* 1986; 204:524–529.

239. Walters JM, et al: Parenteral nutrition by peripheral vein. *Surg Clin North Am* 1981; 61:593–604.

240. Weinsler RL, Krumdieck CL: Death resulting from overzealous total parenteral nutrition: The refeeding syndrome revisited. *Am J Clin Nutr* 1980; 34:393–399.

241. Wentzell RP: *Prevention and Control of Nosocomial Infections.* Baltimore: Williams & Wilkins, 1987, pp 311–312.

242. Winkler B, et al: Relationship of glycerol uptake to plasma glycerol concentration in the normal dog. *Am J Physiol* 1969; 216:191–196.

243. Wolfe RR, et al: Investigation of factors determining the optimal glucose infusion rate in total parenteral nutrition. *Metabolism* 1980; 29:892.

244. Yeung C, et al: Infection rate for single lumen vs. triple lumen subclavian catheters. *Inf Contr Hosp Epidemiol* 1981; 9:154–158.

245. Yoffa D: Supraclavicular subclavian venipuncture and catheterization. *Lancet* 1965; 2:614.

246. Yoshioka K, et al: Influence of total parenteral nutrition (TPN) on nutritional incidence of patients with recurrent cancer. *Gan No Rinsho* 1985; 31:1422–1426.

KEY RECOMMENDED READINGS

For a list of key recommended readings for Chapter 3, see Appendix 2, pp. 288 and 289.

SELF-ASSESSMENT QUESTIONS

Directions. Select the best response to each of the questions or statements below and then enter the corresponding letter in the space provided.

( ) 1. Standard TPN therapy provides an excellent method of long-term (>10 days) supplemental or total nutrition for patients with a nonfunctional gut.

  A. True
  B. False

see p. 110

( ) 2. Standard PPN therapy provides an excellent method of short-term (<10 days) supplemental or total nutrition for patients with a nonfunctional gut.

  A. True
  B. False

see p. 110

( ) 3. Which of the following statements regarding parenteral vs. enteral nutrition therapy is **false?**

  A. Parenteral therapy is associated with a greater incidence of clinical, metabolic, and septic complications.
  B. Parenteral diet administration requires more therapeutic expertise.
  C. Parenteral nutrition therapy is more expensive.
  D. None of the above

see p. 111

( ) 4. A liter of standard TPN solution contains:

  A. $D_{50}W$ 500 cc
  B. Amino acids 8.5%, 500 cc
  C. Routine additives
  D. Optional additives
  E. All of the above

see p. 116

( ) 5. A liter of standard TPN ($D_{50}W$ 500 cc + amino acids 8.5% 500 cc) solution provides approximately_____ kcal.

    A. 200
    B. 400
    C. 500
    D. 1000

see p. 116

( ) 6. A liter of standard TPN ($D_{50}W$ 500 cc + amino acids 8.5% 500 cc) solution provides approximately_____ g of nitrogen.

    A. 7
    B. 20
    C. 30
    D. 40

see p. 116

( ) 7. The ratio of non-protein carbohydrate calories to grams nitrogen of a liter of standard TPN ($D_{50}W$ 500 cc + amino acids 8.5% 500 cc) solution is approximately:

    A. 50:1
    B. 100:1
    C. 150:1
    D. 200:1

see p. 116

( ) 8. To prevent the development of a fatty acid deficiency, fat therapy should provide _____ % of the TPN patient's daily caloric requirement.

    A. <1
    B. 3–5
    C. 10–20
    D. >20

see p. 118

( ) 9. The use of fat to provide >60% of the estimated daily caloric requirement may result in which of the following?

A. Compromised macrophage function
B. Compromised polymorphonuclear cell function
C. Compromised reticuloendothelial cell function
D. All of the above

see p. 118

( ) 10. The incidence of primary catheter infection is higher for a single-lumen central infusion catheter than for a triple-lumen central infusion catheter.

A. True
B. False

see p. 118

( ) 11. Routine TPN therapy should include the administration of at least 500 cc of 20% fat emulsion 3 times per week.

A. True
B. False

see p. 118

( ) 12. The safe infusion of TPN is dependent on the positioning of the central infusion catheter's tip. Which of the following radiologic findings may result in a serious TPN infusion complication?

A. Tip coiled in the innominate vein or superior vena cava
B. Tip in the internal mammary vein
C. Tip in pleural space
D. Tip in the internal jugular vein
E. All of the above

see p. 122

( ) 13. In most clinical situations, the initial adult TPN infusion rate is _____ cc/hr per volumetric pump.

A. 5
B. 20
C. 40
D. 100

see p. 125

( ) 14. A 20% fat emulsion provides approximately _____ kcal/cc.

   A. 1
   B. 2
   C. 3
   D. 4

see p. 118

( ) 15. A TPN infusion of 125 cc/hr administered to an NPO patient can be suddenly discontinued without any risk of hypoglycemia.

   A. True
   B. False

see p. 126

( ) 16. If an NPO patient's TPN infusion is suddenly discontinued, an infusion of _____ at the previous TPN infusion rate should immediately be started to prevent rebound hypoglycemia.

   A. $D_{50}W$
   B. Lactated Ringer's solution
   C. Plasmolyte
   D. $D_{10}NS$

see p. 126

( ) 17. All of the following are common technical complications associated with the insertion of a central infusion catheter, **except:**

   A. Inability to cannulate the vein
   B. Air embolism
   C. Pneumothorax
   D. Bleeding

see p. 127

( ) 18. If an air embolism is suspected, the patient should be placed in the _____ position.

   A. Tendelenburg
   B. lithotomy
   C. Durant
   D. Prone

see p. 128

( ) 19. "Male-female" catheter connections are very dangerous and should not be used in a subclavian (central)
venous catheter infusion system.

    A. True
    B. False

see p. 129

( ) 20. The diagnostic triad for a possible central catheter infection includes all of the following, **except:**

    A. "Plateau" temperature (38.0° to 38.5°C) for 12
to 24 hr
    B. Leucocytosis >10,000 WBC/hpf
    C. Unexplained hyperglycemia (serum glucose
>160 mg/dL)
    D. "Picket fence" temperature pattern

see p. 132

( ) 21. Guidewire exchange of a suspected infected catheter,
in the absence of positive blood cultures and cardiovascular signs of sepsis, is an accepted treatment mo-
dality.

    A. True
    B. False

see p. 132

( ) 22. A catheter tip culture revealing a bacterial colony
count <15 is strongly suggestive of a primary catheter
infection.

    A. True
    B. False

see p. 138

( ) 23. TPN-induced hyperglycemia (serum glucose >160
mg%) is initially treated by immediately decreasing
the TPN infusion rate.

    A. True
    B. False

see p. 134

( ) 24. All of the following statements regarding the "refeed-ing syndrome" are true, **except:**

A. Hypophosphatemia is common.

B. Decreased ventricular stroke work, mean arterial pressure, and congestive cardiomyopathy may occur.

C. The TPN infusion rate should not be increased if the heart rate is greater than 100 beats/min.

D. The TPN infusion rate should be increased 40 cc/hr/day until the required final infusion rate is achieved.

see p. 138

( ) 25. A liter of "concentrated" TPN solution contains $D_{60}W$ or $D_{70}W$, 500 cc, + amino acids _____ % 500 cc.

A. 4.40

B. 4.25

C. 8.50

D. 10.00

see p. 143

( ) 26. A renal failure patient (serum creatinine $>2mg\%$) who cannot be dialyzed and requires fluid restriction should be treated with a TPN solution containing renal failure amino acids.

A. True

B. False

see p. 143

( ) 27. Which of the following renal failure amino acid preparations contains primarily essential amino acids?

A. NephrAmine

B. RenAmin

C. Aminess

D. A and C

E. None of the above

see p. 143

( ) 28. A hepatic failure patient without demonstrable encephalopathy should be treated with a TPN solution containing hepatic failure amino acids.

A. True
B. False

see p. 144

( ) 29. Which of the following is a hepatic failure amino acid preparation?

A. Aminess®
B. Sandostatin®
C. Impact®
D. HepatAmine®

see p. 144

( ) 30. A liter of standard PPN solution contains $D_{20}W$, 500 cc, plus _____ % amino acids, 500 cc.

A. 4.25
B. 5.00
C. 8.50
D. 10.00

see p. 147

( ) 31. On day 1 of PPN therapy, the PPN solution is usually infused at _____ cc/hr.

A. 40
B. 80
C. 100–125
D. None of the above

see p. 149

( ) 32. PPN therapy includes the daily infusion of 20% fat emulsion, 500 cc.

A. True
B. False

see p. 152

( ) 33. A liter of standard PPN ($D_{20}W$ 500 cc + amino acids 10% 500 cc) solution provides approximately _____ kcal and _____ g of nitrogen.

A. 2,000 and 6
B. 1,000 and 7

    C. 400 and 8
    D. 1,000 and 5

see p. 147

( ) 34. The ratio of non-protein carbohydrates to grams nitrogen provided by a liter of standard PPN ($D_{20}W$ 500 cc, and amino acids 10% 500 cc) solution is:

    A. 50:1
    B. 75:1
    C. 100:1
    D. 150:1

see p. 147

( ) 35. All of the following statements regarding ProcalAmine, a "pre-mixed" PPN solution, are true, **EXCEPT:**

    A. Eliminates the problem of solution wastage
    B. Reduces the physician's PPN formulation time
    C. Reduces the pharmacist's PPN mixing time
    D. Provides more calories per liter than a "mixed" PPN solution
    E. Contains glycerol

see p. 153

( ) 36. The final dextrose concentration of a PPN solution cannot exceed 12.5%.

    A. True
    B. False

see p. 155

( ) 37. PPN therapy requires the daily infusion of 3,500 cc (PPN solution 3,000 cc + 20% fat emulsion 500 cc) to provide at least 2,200 kcal and 24 g nitrogen.

    A. True
    B. False

see p. 155

( ) 38. PPN therapy can be safely used to deliver all the daily caloric and protein requirements of the fluid restricted patient (fluid intake limited to <2,000 cc/day).

A. True
B. False

see p. 154

( ) 39. A PPN solution can be successfully used to treat non-fluid-restricted, hepatic failure patients with encephalopathy.

A. True
B. False

see p. 155

( ) 40. When the patient's serum CO_2 <22 mEq/L, the sodium and potassium in the TPN solution should be in the acetate form.

A. True
B. False

see p. 117

( ) 41. When the patient's serum calcium is <8.5 mEq/L, the TPN solution should contain calcium gluconate 9 mEq/L.

A. True
B. False

see p. 117

( ) 42. The potassium content of a TPN solution should not exceed 40 mEq/L. If additional potassium is required, it should be given in intravenous interrupts.

A. True
B. False

see p. 117

( ) 43. A PPN infusion may be discontinued without any risk of rebound hypoglycemia.

A. True
B. False

see p. 152

( ) 44. All of the following are clinical indications for using a special renal failure amino acid preparation, **except:**

A. Dialysis possible

B. Dialysis not possible
C. Serum creatinine >2 mg/dL
D. Abnormal nutritional indices

see p. 143

( ) 45. Which of the following is not routinely added to a TPN or PPN solution?

A. Sodium
B. Trace metals
C. Regular insulin
D. Multivitamins

see pp. 117 and 148

( ) 46. Which of the following are administered daily rather than continuously in each liter of TPN or PPN solution?

A. Multivitamins
B. Amino acids
C. Trace metals
D. A and C

see pp. 117 and 148

( ) 47. A patient with a low serum zinc level is treated by adding elemental zinc, 2–5 mg, to bag 1 of TPN daily in addition to the trace metal supplements routinely added each day to bag 1 of TPN.

A. True
B. False

see p. 136

( ) 48. Prior to starting a TPN infusion, the physician must confirm that the tip of the central infusion catheter is in the superior or inferior vena cava by an expirational chest X-ray.

A. True
B. False

see p. 122

( ) 49. All of the following statements are true regarding PPN therapy, **EXCEPT:**

A. Initial infusion rate of 100–125 cc/hr

B. May be discontinued without a risk of rebound hypoglycemia.
C. Fat therapy provides the major source of calories.
D. Better caloric source than TPN

see p. 112

( ) 50. All of the following increase the risk of air embolism, **except:**
A. "Male-female" connector
B. Luer-Lok connector
C. Reverse Trendelenburg position during catheter insertion or removal
D. Dehydration

see p. 129

ARC/AIDS NUTRITIONAL THERAPY

4

GENERAL DISCUSSION

Investigators are now predicting that nearly 100% of the estimated 12 million patients who have a human immunodeficiency virus (HIV) infection in the world will develop the acquired immune deficiency syndrome. (AIDS).[56, 57] Most persons with AIDS (PWAs) will experience progressive weight loss and malnutrition prior to their death. Because nutritional therapy has clearly been shown to have a beneficial effect on the clinical course and immunologic status of those who are critically-ill in the general population, one must not disregard the potential positive benefits of nutritional therapy in the treatment of PWAs.

As a result of the escalating cost of medical therapy and the current AIDS epidemic, the nutritional management of PWAs must be simple to administer and cost effective. The author has developed nutritional screening criteria to identify those PWAs who would most benefit from nutritional therapy. Because all PWAs differ in their nutritional requirements, diet tolerance, and degree of gut dysfunction, there is no single nutritional therapy that can be routinely used to treat all malnourished PWAs.

The selection of an appropriate oral, enteral, or parenteral diet regimen is crucial in the successful management of these patients. The author has designed specific nutritional therapy algorithms for PWAs with normal and compromised gut function.

Several nutritionists believe that the preservation of nutritional homeostasis may prohibit progressive weight loss, reduce the frequency of secondary infections, augment response to chemotherapy, perhaps retard the deterioration of the immune system, and ultimately improve the overall "quality of life" and "sense of well-being" of PWAs.

Nutritional Deficiencies and Weight Loss

Patients with AIDS-related complex (ARC) and AIDS develop significant nutritional deficiencies and progressive weight loss during the course of their disease.[23, 24, 79, 80, 182, 268, 310] PWAs often have significant potassium, body fat, intracellular water volume, and serum protein depletion.[181-183] In a retrospective review of 50 PWAs, Garcia et al.[129] found that the mean weight loss from preillness usual weight to death was 11.81 ± 7.6 kg. Similarly, O'Sullivan et al.[235] found that PWAs have an average weight loss of 16% from their preillness usual weight prior to death. They discovered that although a large percentage of HIV-infected patients were underweight and malnourished at the time of admission, the majority received only standard diets instead of specialized nutritional supplementation or therapy during the course of their hospitalization.

Malnutrition and Immune Function

Investigators have clearly demonstrated that malnutrition has an adverse effect on immunologic function.* Studies have shown that malnutrition results in

1. A reduction in the total number of T-lymphocytes, helper, and suppressor cells.[64, 68]
2. Impaired cell-mediated[68] and secretory immunity.[284]
3. Reduced complement secretion.[73]
4. Decreased phagocytic function.[173]
5. Decreased killer cell activity.[269]

Furthermore, malnutrition indirectly affects immunologic function by limiting the amount of available amino acid and nucleotide substrates (energy) that are necessary to support cell proliferation.[187, 238]

Malnutrition and Micro-Nutrient Deficiencies

Malnourished patients develop significant deficiencies in minerals, trace metals (iron, copper, zinc, iodine, selenium, magnesium, cobalt, nickel, arsenic, lithium, silicon, and tin)[88, 99, 115, 137] and vitamins (A, C, E, pyridoxine, and folate).[54, 160] These deficiencies adversely effect the AIDS patient's

*References 62, 65–68, 73, 74, 76, 87, 253, 267, 329.

1. Immune function.
2. Recovery from secondary infection.
3. Response to chemotherapy.

Nutritional Therapy and Immune Function

Nutritional repletion plays an important role in the preservation of immunologic function and the successful recovery of critically ill, non-AIDS patients.† It may have a similar affect on PWAs.[49, 50, 119, 181–183, 224] In fact, PWAs treated with a well-designed nutritional therapy regimen early in the course of their disease *may*

1. Experience minimal weight loss.
2. Develop fewer secondary infections.
3. Respond better to chemotherapy.
4. Experience an improved "quality of life" and "sense of well-being."

In addition, aggressive nutritional therapy *may* ultimately retard the immunologic deterioration that occurs in these patients. Unfortunately, at this time there is no clinical data to either support or refute the role of aggressive nutritional therapy in the treatment of PWAs.

Nutritional Therapy For HIV-Infected Patients

At present, there are no specific nutritional therapy guidelines for HIV-infected patients. As a result, many PWAs are eating nontraditional diets and taking expensive food supplements which provide little, if any, nutritional benefit. For example, many AIDS nutritionists are recommending egg-yolk-derived products (e.g., AL-721), megavitamin supplements, dangerous appetite stimulants (e.g., Megace), and inappropriate enteral diets.

In view of the current AIDS crisis and the predicted AIDS epidemic, nutritionists are now faced with the task of designing inexpensive, effective, physiologic nutritional therapy regimens for PWAs. Several important factors must be considered when formulating a nutritional therapy regimen for these patients. These factors include

1. Epidemiologic and economic data.
2. Psychosocial status.

†References 12, 33, 34, 140, 141, 162, 198, 253.

3. Etiologies for gut dysfunction.
4. Nutrient requirements.
5. Therapeutic goal.
6. Treatment options.
7. Types of diets.
8. Specific therapeutic regimens.

EPIDEMIOLOGIC AND ECONOMIC DATA

Epidemiologic Data

Infection with HIV and AIDS are now a major cause of morbidity and mortality in the United States.[56, 57, 89, 148, 157] Of all adult cases, 73% were in homosexual or bisexual men. Seventeen percent of the adult cases were heterosexuals with a history of intravenous drug abuse. The remaining 10% were hemophiliacs, transfusion-associated cases, or cases resulting from heterosexual contact with an infected person. In a few instances, the means of transmission was unknown.[89]

Prevalence estimates for HIV infection indicate that between 10% and 70% of homosexual and bisexual men are infected.[89] Among women, the highest risk groups are intravenous drug abusers and those who have had heterosexual contact with a member of a high-risk group.[148, 157] Pediatric AIDS is acquired perinatally or through the transfusion of blood products.

Recently, the World Health Organization (WHO) estimated that as many as 10 million people worldwide are infected with HIV. According to WHO records, as many as 800,000 people have developed AIDS since 1981 and nearly half of these individuals have died. It also predicts that 15 to 20 million people worldwide will be HIV positive by the year 2000.

Economic Data

The United States Public Health Service Planning Conference on AIDS has projected that by 1991 nearly 54,000 U.S. citizens will die as a result of AIDS.[56, 57, 89, 148, 157] By comparison, there were 2.1 million deaths from all causes during 1986.[34] The medical costs (excluding aggressive nutritional therapy) for the 270,000 AIDS cases diagnosed between 1981 and the end of 1991 in the United States are projected to be $22 billion.[34]

The economic impact of AIDS will not be evenly distributed. Cities such as San Francisco and New York (where approximately 10,000 AIDS cases were diagnosed as of 1987) will bear most of the burden.[330] By mid-1987 approximately 500,000 persons in the New York City metropolitan area were infected with the AIDS virus. Not only did this challenge available hospital space, it also forced the development of long-term home and hospice care programs.[330]

PSYCHOSOCIAL STATUS

Factors Affecting the Psychosocial Milieu

The psychosocial status of AIDS patients is affected by the physical aspects of the disease.[168, 230, 232, 242, 275, 276, 287, 307, 337] The PWA's psychosocial milieu is influenced by several factors: (1) physical, owing to the effects of the disease and related opportunistic infections; (2) psychological, owing to the emotional impact of rapid physical breakdown, the possibility of severe economic losses, and the realization that one is faced with a terminal illness; and (3) social, owing to the emotional response of relatives and friends and their subsequent contagion fears on learning of the AIDS diagnosis.[28, 207]

Factors Affecting Daily Activities

The daily activities of the individuals with AIDS may be compromised in many ways. An HIV infection can cause several systemic problems, such as

- Diarrhea
- Fatigue
- Weakness
- Weight loss
- Cachexia
- Anorexia
- Night sweats
- General malaise.

Each of these can adversely affect the PWA's ability to work effectively or at all.[28, 159]

The central nervous system (CNS) is frequently affected by an HIV infection.* Patients with a CNS HIV infection often experience

- Memory loss
- Dementia

*References 168, 207, 230, 275, 276, 287, 307, 337.

- Dysequilibrium[207]
- Headaches
- Seizures
- Tremors
- Blurred vision
- Incontinence
- Dysphagia
- Confusion
- Impaired cognitive ability
- Visual, auditory, gustatory, and olfactory problems[28, 159]

Because of these CNS-related problems, PWAs are often physically unable to care for themselves.

Shock, denial, anxiety, and even social withdrawal may follow the AIDS diagnosis.[28, 159] Because of the uncertainty implied by this diagnosis, the guilt of an exposed prior lifestyle, and the fear of impending doom, PWAs may become depressed.[95] The newly diagnosed "closet" homosexual may also fear the response of his family and friends on learning of his sexual orientation. Similarly, an HIV infected intravenous drug abuser may fear rejection and prejudice.[28]

In summary, the systemic CNS and psychological effects of an HIV infection can adversely affect the PWAs' daily activities, response to medical therapy,[28, 95] and eventually, their nutrient intake. The nutritionist must therefore consider the AIDS patient's psychosocial milieu when designing a nutritional therapy regimen.[28]

ETIOLOGIES FOR GUT DYSFUNCTION
Infections

Patients with AIDS are immunosuppressed and consequently vulnerable to infection by a variety of microorganisms, including fungi, viruses, protozoa, mycobacteria, and bacteria (Table 4–1).[33, 39, 159, 264] The symptoms and physical manifestations of the various AIDS-related infections are discussed in Table 4–2. These infections frequently involve the gastrointestinal tract (Table 4–3).* Depending on the level of involvement and the severity of the infection, individuals may experience significant nutritional deficiencies.[23, 24, 79, 80, 182, 268, 310]

*References 5, 6, 13, 16, 82, 100, 131, 134, 202, 257.

TABLE 4–1.

AIDS-Related Infections*

Infecting Organism	Type of Infection
Viruses	
Cytomegalovirus	Pneumonia, disseminated infection, retinitis, encephalitis
Epstein-Barr	B cell lymphoproliferative disorders, Burkitt's lymphoma, oral hairy leukoplakia
Herpes simplex	Recurrent, severe, localized infection
Herpes zoster	Localized or disseminated infection
Papovavirus	Progressive multifocal leukoencephalopathy
Fungi	
Candida albicans	Mucocutaneous infection, esophagitis, disseminated infection
Cryptococcus neoformans	Meningitis, disseminated infection
Histoplasma capsulatum	Disseminated infection
Coccidioides immitis	Disseminated infection
Petriellidium boydii	Pneumonia
Aspergillus	Invasive pulmonary infection with potential dissemination
Protozoa	
Pneumocystis carinii	Pneumonia, retinal infection
Toxoplasma gondii	Encephalitis
Cryptosporidium	Enteritis
Isospora belli	Enteritis
Mycobacteria	
Mycobacterium avium-intracellulare	Disseminated infection
Mycobacterium tuberculosis	Disseminated infection
Bacteria	
Nocardia	Pneumonia, disseminated infection
Legionella	Pneumonia
Streptoccus pneumonia	Pneumonia, disseminated infection
Hemophilus influenza, type B	Pneumonia, disseminated infection
Salmonella	Gastroenteritis, disseminated infection
Campylobacter	Enteritis

*Adapted from Rubin RH: Acquired immunodeficiency syndrome, in Rubenstein E, Federman D (eds): *Scientific American Medicine.* New York: Scientific American, Inc, 1987.

TABLE 4–2.
Symptoms and Physical Manifestations of AIDS-Related Infections*

Infection	Symptoms and Manifestations
Candida albicans	
Oral (thrush)	Loss of appetite, white plaques, mouth discomfort or change in taste
Pharyngeal	Dysphagia, sore throat
Esophageal	Substernal burning-type pain, difficulty swallowing
Proctal	Rectal pain, weeping lesions (without plaques), pruritus
Cryptococcus neoformans	
Meningitis	Fever, severe headache, obtundation, stiff neck, change in mental status, untoward side effects related to antibiotics
Cryptosporidium enteritis	Severe watery diarrhea (up to 15 to 20 L/day), weakness, abdominal cramping, fever, nausea, vomiting
Cytomegalovirus	Blindness or visual loss (retinitis), fever, fatigue/severe malaise, weight loss, facial edema (secondary to adrenalitis)
Herpes simplex	Weeping skin lesions (oral, perirectal), rectal bleeding, rectal discharge
Herpes zoster (shingles)	Vesicular skin lesions along dermatomes, pain
Mycobacterium avium-intracellulare	Fever, severe weight loss/cachexia, abdominal pain, diarrhea, malabsorption, antibiotic side effects
Pneumocystis carinii pneumonia	Fever, chills, night sweats, cough with/without sputum production, dyspnea, antibiotic side effects, weight loss, weakness
Progressive multifocal leukoencephalopathy	Progressive weakness and dementia, speech problems, forgetfulness, perceptual problems, visual problems, incontinence

*Adapted from Hughes A, et al: *AIDS Home Care and Hospice Manual.* AIDS home care and hospice program, San Francisco; San Francisco Visiting Nurse Association, 1987.

TABLE 4-3.

AIDS-Related Alimentary Tract Infections

Anatomic Location	Infection
Oropharynx and esophagus	Candidiasis
	Ulcerations and a maculopapular rash probably due to HTLV-III/LAV
	Ulcerations due to HSV I and II
	Hairy leukoplakia due to Epstein-Barr virus and papilloma virus
	Kaposi's sarcoma
Stomach and small bowel	Gastric ulcerations probably due to HTLV-III/LAV
	Ulcerations due to cytomegalovirus
	Kaposi's sarcoma
Colon and rectum	Cytomegalovirus ulceration and perforation
	Cryptosporidiosis
	Isosporiasis
	Anal and cloacogenic carcinoma
	Mycobacterium avium-intracellulare colitis
	"Gay bowel syndrome" with bacteremia
	Lymphogranuloma venereum (chlamydial) proctitis
	HSV I and II proctitis

Fungal Infections

Patients frequently develop oral candidiasis (thrush).[177] In one study, 94% of the patients had oral candidiasis.[22] Other oral infections include aphthous and infections ulcers and mucositis.[16, 22, 243] Patients with thrush, ulcers, and mucositis may experience a burning sensation or dysphagia with food ingestion[19]; consequently, their nutrient intake is significantly reduced.

Viral Infections

The mucosa of both the small and large bowel is a major target for the HIV.[184, 268] Patients with an intestinal HIV infection develop severe diarrhea, which is frequently refractory to aggressive antidiarrheal therapy. Because of the voluminous diarrhea (3 to 8 L/day), these patients develop electrolyte imbalance, dehydration, and trace metal deficiencies.[28] Studies suggest that male homosexual PWAs may have a greater tendency to develop refractory diarrhea because of their increased exposure to gastrointestinal pathogens[184, 268] than female homosexual PWAs.

In addition to the HIV infection, PWAs can develop cytomegalovirus (CMV),[121, 178, 217, 331] HSV I or II, and various enterovirus intestinal infections. Those with a CMV intestinal infection have gastrointestinal symptoms similar to patients with inflammatory bowel disease.[81] Because of this, patients with possible inflammatory bowel disease should be questioned regarding their risk for an HIV infection.[27]

Bacterial Infections

Patients with AIDS develop diarrhea because of a bacterial or protozoan intestinal infection. The most common bacterial infections include *Shigella, Salmonella, Campylobacter,* unusual *E. Coli,* enterococci,[335] and *Mycobacterium avium-intracellulare.*[134, 263, 306]

Parasitic Infections

The most common parasitic intestinal infection is cryptosporidiosis.[216, 221, 227, 233, 303, 331] Patients with a *Cryptosporidium* infection of the gut often have severe, profuse, secretory diarrhea that is refractory to chemotherapy and antidiarrheal therapy.* Unless successfully treated, these patients rapidly become dehydrated, develop electrolyte imbalance and trace metal deficiencies, and become severely malnourished.[285, 299] Eventually, they die from dehydration, electrolyte abnormalities, and malnutrition.[221]

Malignancy

Patients with AIDS may develop alimentary tract neoplasms. Kaposi's sarcoma (KS) is the most common gastrointestinal tract tumor found in PWAs. Individuals with alimentary tract KS lesions have a significantly greater mortality than patients with no KS lesions.[80] Oral and esophageal KS lesions may cause pain and dysphagia. Small bowel and colonic KS lesions can cause complete or incomplete intestinal obstruction. Intestinal mucosal KS lesions often cause intractable diarrhea and subsequent malabsorption.

Alimentary tract neoplasms often adversely affect nutrient intake. Depending on the size and location of the tumor, gastro-

*References 30, 86, 91, 178, 192, 220, 247, 316.

intestinal functions may be severely compromised. Consequently, PWAs with gastrointestinal tract tumors must be treated with special enteral and parenteral diets to prevent progressive nutritional deterioration.

Nonspecific Enteropathy

Patients with AIDS may develop a nonspecific enteropathy that cannot be explained by the presence of an infectious agent or tumor. This NSE is caused by a pathologic process in the lamina propria of the small bowel or the colon. PWAs with diarrhea (refractory to chemotherapy), D-xylose malabsorption, and steatorrhea frequently have histologic changes in their jejunal and rectal mucosa that are consistent with an NSE. Because their gastrointestinal tract lining is severely damaged,[184] the ability of these patients to absorb important nutrients and to maintain nutritional homeostasis is severely compromised.[99]

NUTRIENT REQUIREMENTS
Body Composition

Body composition studies have shown that the body cell mass of most PWAs is significantly depleted.[183] One study revealed that, despite their successful response to chemotherapy and subsequent hospital discharge, several PWAs failed to replete their body cell mass, and remained malnourished. This suggests that the malnutrition seen in PWAs may be resistant to therapy and that it may contribute to their deaths.[184]

The rate and extent of weight loss may determine the PWA's life expectancy. The cause for the PWA's life-threatening weight loss has not been clearly identified. Chlebowski[77] has suggested that it may involve a complex interaction among simple starvation, malabsorption, and inability of the body's cells to utilize nutrients.

AIDS Malnutrition

Patients with inadequate nutrient intake may become malnourished. There are two types of malnutrition: (1) protein malnutrition, which occurs when the diet is deficient in protein, *and* (2) protein-calorie malnutrition (PCM), which occurs as a consequence of general starvation and the inadequate intake of both protein and calories.

Protein Malnutrition

Protein malnutrition causes muscle atrophy, delayed wound healing, prolonged ventilatory dependence, impaired immunocompetence, delayed bone callus formation, and abnormal red cell function. It may occur as a result of chronic diarrhea, renal dysfunction, infection, hemorrhage, trauma, or burns. Protein malnutrition is characterized by reduced serum albumin and transferrin levels, decreased serum iron-binding capacity, and delayed cellular immunity. Weight loss is inconsistent and may not be recognized because of fluid retention. The set of clinical findings and laboratory findings that occur as a result of protein malnutrition are described as the kwashiorkor syndrome.

Protein-Calorie Malnutrition

Protein-calorie malnutrition occurs as a result of general starvation. This form of malnutrition is characterized by bradycardia, hypothermia, reduced basal metabolism, depletion of subcutaneous fat and tissue turgor, and the development of wrinkled skin. Patients with protein-calorie malnutrition consistently lose weight and require intense nutritional therapy. The set of clinical findings and laboratory findings that occur as a result of protein-calorie malnutrition are described as the marasmus syndrome.

Effects of Starvation

Patients with AIDS usually suffer from PCM.[183, 184] It occurs as a result of either (1) the effect of the HIV infection on gut function (absorption) *or* (2) inadequate nutrient intake secondary to HIV-induced infections before or during hospitalization.

It is well known that starvation causes villous atrophy and the reduction of intestinal enzyme production. Kotler et al.[184] have shown that an HIV infection can result in villous destruction and altered gut function. Villous atrophy or destruction causes decreased absorptive surface area and impaired digestive capacity.[6] Patients suffering from either of these problems become progressively more malnourished. Unless successfully treated, they eventually die from a combination of both malnutrition and HIV-induced infection.[181-183]

Metabolic and Physiologic Effects of Secondary Infections

Patients with AIDS frequently suffer from secondary infections which increase their metabolic requirements and compromise their nutrient intake. Several complex, predictable metabolic and physiologic responses occur in the presence of infection. Many of these induce nutritional losses from body stores. The classic metabolic effects of sepsis include weight loss, marked reduction in muscle mass, decreasing serum albumin level, and negative nitrogen balance.[214] If diarrhea is a part of the symptom complex, the speed and magnitude of nutritional losses are usually greater than those seen in an infectious process where diarrhea is not involved.[25]

Metabolic Effects of Sepsis

In sepsis, the process of muscle proteolysis is exaggerated. Muscle is catabolized in response to the body's demand for energy. Instead of sequentially using glucose, fat, and finally amino acids, as in the milder state of starvation, energy production becomes progressively protein based.[59] This promotes the rapid development of negative nitrogen balance.

If the excessive protein catabolism induced by sepsis continues unabated, the patient's amino acid supply is rapidly exhausted. This consequently weakens the body's ability to defend itself against infection or to repair damaged organs and tissues.[26] The acquisition of subsequent infections further compromise the PWA's defense mechanism, until eventually a life-threatening deficit occurs. During a febrile illness, several anabolic processes occur. One of the most important is the synthesis of proteins to maintain the function of phagocytic neutrophils, monocytes, macrophages, and various subsets of lymphocytes. A great variety of proteins are needed to maintain the host's defense, especially immunoglobulin and antimicrobial factors such as interferon, lysozyme, transferrin, lactoferrin, coagulation components, and various acute-phase proteins. Some of these proteins are synthesized from free amino acids mobilized from muscle protein. Unfortunately, however, the wasting effects of illness often tend to overshadow the anabolic activity that creates important host defense proteins.[25, 26]

In prolonged sepsis, complications may occur that lead to immunocompetence of physiologically controlled defense mechanisms and cellular function. Because PWAs often suffer from protracted sepsis, they frequently experience major derangements of acid-base balance, severe depletion of body nutrients, alteration in respiration and cardiovascular function, hypotension, tissue anoxia, and cardiac failure.[26] These derangements may respond to appropriate exogenous metabolic support, provided that (1) the septic process is adequately controlled *and* (2) the patient's nutritional status is not critically depleted.[59]

Immunologic Effects of Protein-Calorie Malnutrition

Studies of undernourished children and adults have demonstrated that malnutrition impairs immunocompetence. PCM is associated with progressive changes in

1. Cell-mediated immunity.
2. Neutrophilic bactericidal function.
3. The complement system.
4. The secretory IgA antibody response.[64, 69–71, 75, 191]

Protein-calorie malnutrition causes the central organs of the immune system to atrophy in children, particularly the thymus and peripheral tissues, such as lymph nodes, tonsils, and spleen.[229]

Cutaneous hypersensitivity responses to common microbial antigens are absent or reduced in PCM. There is also a deficiency of thymus-dependent T-lymphocytes.[76, 260] Patients with PCM have a marked reduction in their proportion of T-4 helper cells and a moderately reduced proportion of T-8 cytotoxic, suppressor cells.[76] Total hemolytic complement activity, as well as serum levels of C3, factor B, and other components of the complement system are reduced in PWAs with PCM. Also, polyclonal hyperimmunoglobulinemia is common in this group of patients.[76]

The multiple infections and severe weight loss common in PWAs resemble those seen in PCM.[146] Patients with AIDS and children with PCM suffer from multiple opportunistic infections.[62, 67–69, 73, 231] Both types of patients have an increased incidence of KS lesions and diffuse, undifferentiated B cell lymphomas which are histologically similar to Burkitt's lymphoma.[146]

The pattern of immunodeficiency in PWAs and children with PCM is also similar. In PCM, a reduction of cell-mediated immunity particularly affects the T-lymphocytes. In PWAs, there is a consistent decrease in the ratio of circulating T-helper to suppressor cells. Both groups also have lymphopenia and pronounced lymphocyte depletion in both their lymph nodes and spleen.[146]

Researchers have hypothesized that PWAs who are subclinically immunodeficient as a result of existing malnutrition, or of deficiencies in micronutrients, trace minerals, vitamins, or amino acids, or a combination of both, may rapidly develop full-blown

AIDS once infected. They have also suggested that well-nourished PWAs may be symptom-free and only suffer from chronic lymphadenopathy following the successful treatment of their infection.[163] Studies have also shown that malnourished, HIV-infected individuals with suboptimal immunity are more susceptible to opportunistic infections.[163]

Pre-existing or additional nutritional defects may further compromise the PWA's immune function, aggravate the effects of opportunistic infections, or predispose the PWA to further infectious processes. When this occurs, it potentiates the vicious cycle of recurrent infections and eventually the patient's death.[99] Because of this, it has been suggested that restoration of nutritional homeostasis may be a useful adjunct in the treatment of PWAs.[163]

Glutamine

Glutamine is the most abundant amino acid in both whole blood and the intracellular free amino acid pool. In conjunction with alanine, glutamine transports more than half of the circulating amino acid nitrogen.[290, 295, 298] Glutamine, rather than glucose, is the major oxidative substrate for the small intestine.[294–296] It is a major energy source for all body cells.[289–291, 293, 295, 296, 298] As part of its role in regulating nitrogen metabolism, glutamine is actively broken down in the small intestine.[289–291, 293, 295, 296, 298] It is avidly consumed by replicating cells such as fibroblasts, lymphocytes, tumor cells and intestinal epithelial cells. The concentration of glutamine in whole blood and skeletal muscle decreases markedly following injury or during catabolic disease states.[289, 291, 293, 295, 296]

Glutamine metabolism by the intestine generates alanine, which is used by the liver for gluconeogenesis and by the kidney for ammoniagenesis. Starving and ketoacidosis stimulate the release of glutamine from intact muscle and its uptake by the kidney. It is theorized that during prolonged starvation the kidney uses glutamine for gluconeogenesis. The diminished levels of circulating glutamine during stress or critical illness suggest that glutamine uptake is also accelerated in other tissues.[289, 291, 293–295, 297–299]

The preservation of the integrity of the small bowel mucosa, and possibly that of the stomach, may require adequate amounts of glutamine from either exogenous or endogenous sources. This requirement appears to increase during critical illness because of the increased intestinal metabolism of gluta-mine.[289–291, 293, 296, 298, 299]

Accelerated protein catabolism during infection and critical illness is associated with a diminished muscle glutamine pool, a reduced plasma glutamine level, and possibly, increased intestinal glutamine utilization. In view of this and the fact that glutamine is the preferential energy source for the small bowel mucosa, exogenous glutamine supplementation, either enterally or parenterally, is extremely important for metabolically stressed patients. Consequently, PWAs should receive enteral or parenteral diets fortified with glutamine to maintain the integrity of the small bowel mucosa and to enhance the absorption of nutrients.

Arginine

Arginine is considered a semi-essential amino acid. Although the body is normally able to synthesize arginine in sufficient amounts, under certain conditions, dietary arginine may be indispensable for optimal growth in certain adult mammals. Of therapeutic significance are the studies that document the need for dietary arginine following trauma and injury and its beneficial role in improving wound healing and reducing nitrogen losses.[20] These and other important metabolic activities of arginine are listed as follows:

- Required for protein synthesis.
- Source for the transport, storage, and excretion of nitrogen.
- Potent hormonal secretagogue.
- Required for the synthesis of creatine and polyamines.
- Protects against ammonia intoxication via urea synthesis.
- Thymotropic activity.

Arginine is obtained from the diet and by endogenous synthesis which is closely linked with the urea cycle enzymes of both the liver and kidney. Very little arginine is released by the liver because of high liver arginase activity. The kidney, however, has lower arginase activity and is therefore able to generate arginine from the uptake of citrulline released by the gut. The arginine is then released into the circulation for tissue protein synthesis. Arginine is absorbed in the intestine by an active transport system which is sodium dependent and substrate specific. Because it is one of the least toxic amino acids, high doses of dietary arginine have been well tolerated in humans.[325]

More recently, the immune and metabolic effects of arginine have been evaluated in a randomized prospective trial of 30 cancer patients undergoing major operations. Patients who received enteral diets supplemented with arginine were shown to have significant enhancement in T-lymphocyte activation to concanavalin A and phytohemagglutinin and an increase in mean CD4 phenotype (Figs 4–1 and 4–2). These immune stimulation responses appear to be distinct from effects on nitrogen balance.[92] From this research, supplemental arginine was shown to have enhanced immunocompetence in patients whose cellular immunity was impaired by the metabolic stress of illness and surgery.

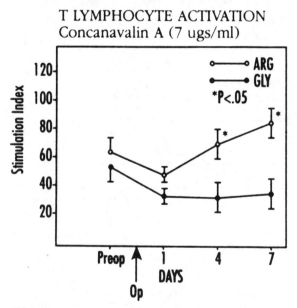

T LYMPHOCYTE ACTIVATION
Concanavalin A (7 ugs/ml)

FIG 4–1.
T-lymphocyte activation. In both groups, T-lymphocyte activation to Concanavalin A decreased significantly from the preoperative period to postoperative day 1. However, in the arginine group (ARG) there was a rapid rise back to normal levels on days 4 and 7, whereas mean values remained low in the glycine (GLY) group (mean ± SEM).

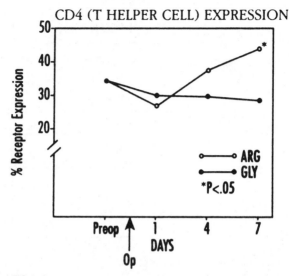

FIG 4–2.
CD4 (T-helper cell) expression. On day 17, mean CD4 (T-helper cell) expression increased significantly in the arginine group (ARG) compared with the glycine group (GLY).

Nucleotides

Nucleotides are precursors of deoxyribonucleic acid (DNA) and ribonucleic acid (RNA) and are involved in almost all living processes. As a carrier of genetic information, DNA serves as a template for the formation of RNA. Most RNA molecules, in turn, direct the synthesis of cellular proteins.

Nucleotides have three main components (Fig 4–3):

- Pentose sugar.
- Nitrogenous base.
- One or more phosphate groups.

The pentose sugar can either be ribose, found in RNA, or 2-deoxyribose, found in DNA. The nitrogenous bases are the pu-

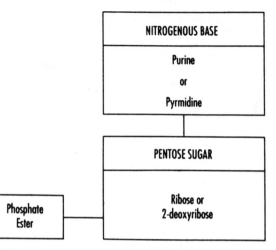

FIG 4–3.
Three main components of nucleotides.

rines, adenine and guanine, and pyrimidines, cytosine, thymine, and uracil (Fig 4–4).

In addition to serving as the structural units of DNA and RNA, nucleotides participate in a number of metabolic reactions fundamental to cellular activity. Adenosine triphosphate (ATP), the major substance used by organisms for the transfer of chemical energy is an adenine nucleotide. Adenine is also a component of the coenzymes nicotinamide adenine dinucleotide, flavin adenine dinucleotide, and coenzyme A. These coenzymes are important in carbohydrate, protein, and lipid synthesis.

The body obtains nucleotides from dietary sources or from biosynthesis in various tissues, such as the liver. The large polynucleotides are absorbed in the intestine, broken down into the nitrogenous bases, taken up by the cells, and converted to nucleotides. The purine and pyrimidine bases are constantly being converted into RNA, DNA, or other nucleotides and are reutilized by means of salvage pathways, or degraded and excreted.

Certain rapidly growing cells, such as T-lymphocytes and intestinal epithelial cells, appear to lack the ability to synthesize nu-

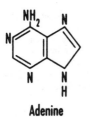

Adenine

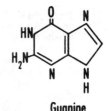

PURINES

Guanine

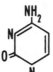

Cytosine

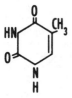

Thymine

PYRIMIDINES

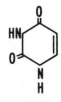

Uracil

FIG 4–4.
Major purine and pyrimidine bases.

cleotides. These cells depend on the salvage pathway or dietary sources for sufficient amounts of nucleotides to be able to synthesize proteins and proliferate.[259, 263]

Based on experimental data,[26] it is believed that these salvage/dietary sources are inadequate during severe metabolic stress, such as trauma, burns, and sepsis, thereby contributing to the immune dysfunction present in these conditions.

Although nucleotides were previously not considered essential nutrients, recent investigations have demonstrated their importance in maintaining cellular immune responses. Initially, transplant patients receiving total parenteral nutrition, which is nucleotide-free, were observed to have fewer episodes of organ rejections. This decreased allograft rejection was thought to be a result of the immunosuppressive effects of a nucleotide-free diet, which has since been confirmed by animal studies.[2]

Nucleotide-free diets have also been reported to decrease delayed hypersensitivity responses,[187] resistance to infections,[111] and interleukin-2 production.[320] These immunosuppressive effects are directly related to the unique metabolic requirements of T-lymphocytes for nucleotides, which appear to be necessary for T-cell maturation and expression of phenotype makers. The addition of nucleotides to enteral and parenteral formulations, most of which are nucleotide-free, may have therapeutic applications for patients who are immunocompromised as a result of metabolic stress or illness and at risk of developing infectious complications, for example, PWAs.

Trace Metals

The relationship of individual trace metals to physiologic responses in PWAs is not well documented. The importance of trace metals to non-AIDS patients is, however, fairly well understood.* In the following six subsections, the importance of several vital trace metals in the general, non-AIDS patient population are briefly discussed.

Selenium Deficiency

Selenium deficiency has been associated with fungal infection, an increased risk of neoplastic diseases, anemia, and congestive heart failure.* While a pure selenium deficiency causes few clinical manifestations, it may predispose the intestinal mucosa to injury by other agents.[184] Diminished T-cell numbers have been reported in patients receiving total parenteral nutrition without selenium supplementation. Low selenium levels, along with low vitamin E and beta carotene or retinal intake, appear to contribute to an increased risk of death from cancer in one study.[266]

Dworkin et al.[99, 100] found that PWAs had significantly lower levels of blood selenium than healthy, non-AIDS patients. The levels were low in both the plasma and the red blood cells, the latter suggesting long-term selenium depletion. The diminished selenium levels occurred in PWAs regardless of the presence or absence of diarrhea, bowel pathogens, or malabsorption. There was a strong positive correlation between plasma selenium and serum albumin, both of which were diminished in PWAs. Since se-

*References 15, 18, 100, 117, 119, 151, 162, 176, 195, 197, 213, 228, 246, 272, 273, 319, 336, 343.

*References 50, 84, 113, 124, 147, 165, 175, 212.

lenium is bound to non-albumin proteins, the low selenium level was not thought to be the result of low albumin levels.[100]

Zinc Deficiency

Zinc deficiency in non-AIDS patients with primary hypogammaglobulinemia is associated with impaired proliferative response to mitogens and low levels of thymic hormones.[47, 135, 136] In vitro, lymphocytes display a decreased response to mitogens and antigens and depressed T-killer cell activity. In addition, zinc-deficient patients have diminished humoral immunity, suppressed thymic hormone activity, and impaired, delayed, cutaneous hypersensitivity reactions.[25, 26, 70, 248, 340] Patients with AIDS frequently have a zinc deficiency.[47, 109, 110] Shoemaker et al.[281] discovered that PWAs with chronic diarrhea frequently had either low or borderline serum zinc levels. Because of this and the immunologic importance of zinc within the non-AIDS patient population, nutritionists believe that PWAs should receive zinc supplements.[105]

Copper Deficiency

A copper deficiency is associated with an increased incidence of infection, depressed reticuloendothelial cell function, and reduced microbicidal activity of the granulocytes.[76, 219, 279]

Chromium and Molybdenum Deficiencies

Chromium, an important trace metal,* is a vital component of the glucose tolerance factor. During the hypermetabolic phase of acute illness or injury, glucose metabolism (serum clearance) is normally reduced. In the presence of a chromium deficiency, serum glucose tolerance factor is reduced and subsequently the metabolism of glucose is reduced during the hypermetabolic phase. Clinically, a chromium deficiency results in impaired glucose tolerance, disturbance in carbohydrate and lipid metabolism, neuropathy, and weight loss. Molybdenum, like selenium, is an essential component of several enzyme systems.* Clinically, a molybdenum deficiency results in amino acid intolerance, irritability, lethargy, coma, and headache.

Iron Deficiency

Iron deficiency is associated with impaired lymphocyte response to mitogens and decreased neutrophil bactericidal capacity.[35, 65, 74, 75] Patients with an iron deficiency suffer from increasing fatigue, headache, anorexia[150] or capricious appetite,

*References 8, 50, 84, 98, 147, 155, 166, 167, 175, 212, 251.

heartburn, palpitation, dyspnea, pedal edema, neuralgic pains, vasomotor disturbances, and paresthesia.[17, 37, 338]

Iodine Deficiency

Iodine has been shown to play an important role in the microbial activity of polymorphonuclear leukocytes. In hypothyroid patients, this activity was significantly reduced. Iodine is an integral component of the thyroid hormones thyroxine and triiodothyronine. These hormones have an important metabolic role. An iodine deficiency causes thyroid enlargement (goiter) and compromised metabolism. Because of its role in the microbicidal activity of the polymorphonuclear cells and metabolism, iodine appears to be an important trace metal for PWAs.

Lipids

Laboratory animals deprived of fatty acids develop lymphoid atrophy and have a reduced antibody response to antigen stimulation.[24, 63, 68, 75, 76] In contrast, an excess rather than a deficiency in certain lipids is the source of most lipid-related immunologic abnormalities in humans. In view of this, oral fat supplements or intravenous fat emulsion therapy should not provide greater than 50% of the PWA's daily caloric requirement.*

Recently, there has been considerable interest in the effect of omega-3 fatty acids on immune function. Dietary lipids perform a number of important physical, nutritional, and biochemical functions. Recent developments have focused on the structural and regulatory functions of fatty acids, specifically the polyunsaturated fatty acids (PUFAs). Because fatty acids can be incorporated directly into the phospholipid molecules of cell membranes, they can alter the ability of the cells to interact and to release regulatory substances.

Polyunsaturated Fatty Acids

The essential PUFAs can be classified into two major families: omega-6 and omega-3 fatty acids. The families are defined by the location of the first double bond from the terminal methyl end of the carbon chains. Linoleic acid is an example of the omega-6 PUFAs, as alpha-linolenic acid is for the omega-3 PUFAs. Vegetable oils such as corn, safflower, sunflower, and soybean oils are good sources of linoleic acid. Vegetable sources of alpha-linolenic acid are more limited and include linseed, canola, walnut, and soybean oils. Cold water fish are a rich source of omega-3 fatty

*References 136, 193, 198, 201, 205, 206, 288.

acids, specifically eicosapentaenoic acid (EPA) and docosa-hexaenoic acid (DHA), which are normally derived by desatura-tion and elongation of alpha-linolenic acid.

Following digestion and absorption,[169] dietary fatty acids may be oxidized for energy sources; stored in adipose tissue; or further metabolized by desaturation, elongation, and oxygenation to vari-ous long-chain PUFAs and selectively incorporated into cells. The omega-6 and omega-3 fatty acids differ in structure and metabo-lism, as well as in biochemical and physiological effects (Fig 4–5).

Linoleic acid is desaturated and elongated to form arachidonic acid. Arachidonic acid is a precursor to the synthesis of ei-cosanoids, specifically the series-2 prostaglandins and series-4 leukotrienes. Eicosanoids are potent biochemical mediators of

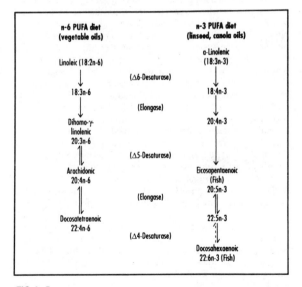

FIG 4–5.
Metabolism, desaturation and elongation of dietary linoleic and linolenic acid in humans.

cell-to-cell communication which are involved in inflammation, infection, tissue injury, and immune system modulation.

Delta-6 desaturase, the key enzyme that converts linoleic acid to arachidonic acid, also regulates the conversion of alpha-linolenic acid to EPA. EPA is a precursor to the synthesis of a less potent series of eicosanoids, the series-3 prostaglandins and series-5 leukotrienes. These biochemical mediators compete with or inhibit the effects of the eicosanoids produced by the omega-6 fatty acids. However, because delta-6 desaturase is a rate-limiting enzyme, alpha-linolenic acid may not be efficient in forming EPA and DHA. Therefore, a dietary source of EPA, such as fish oils, is required to favorably manipulate eicosanoid production.

Effects of Polyunsaturated Fatty Acids on the Immune System

Efficient functioning of the immune system appears to be dependent on a balance of eicosanoid production between the omega-6 and omega-3 fatty acids. Eicosanoids appear to modulate numerous events involving both cell-mediated and humoral immunity and can be synthesized in varying amounts by all immune cells, especially macrophages and monocytes. Diets high in omega-6 fatty acids have been shown to suppress immune function by inhibiting mitogenesis due to increased prostaglandin E_2 synthesis which inhibits T-cell proliferation.[67-69]

In a study of the metabolic effects and immune responses of lipid type of postburn nutritional support, burned guinea pigs were enterally fed diets identical in fat content but with varied fat sources: safflower oil, pure linoleic acid, and fish oil. On completion of the study, the animals receiving fish oil as the lipid source had significantly better weight, lower metabolic expenditure, and improved immune responses than the animals fed either linoleic acid or safflower oil (Fig. 4-6). These results are attributed to the effect of dietary lipids on eicosanoid production following burn injury.[2, 3]

In another study, the effects of various PUFAs on rat sepsis mortality were evaluated using a cecal ligation and puncture (CLP) model. Rats were fed diets of 70% carbohydrate, 28% protein, and 2% fat by weight with the fat source as either coconut, safflower, corn, or menhaden (fish) oils. After 3 months of feeding, CLP was performed and those rats surviving 96 hours after the CLP were sacrificed. A direct relationship between mortality and the ratio of arachidonic acid to EPA was noted on determin-

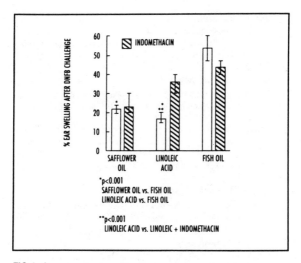

FIG 4–6.
Cell-mediated immunity and opsonic index of burned animals.

ing the liver PUFA content, with mortality increasing as the ratio increased.[58, 59]

These and other observations suggest that cell-to-cell communication can be modulated by altering dietary PUFA composition and that adverse effects of current fat formulations may be occurring in sepsis. Patients who are immunocompromised from illness or injury may derive therapeutic benefits from a nutritional formulation which provides a balance of omega-6 and omega-3 fatty acids.

Vitamins

The relationship of individual vitamins to physiologic response in PWAs is not well documented. The importance of several key vitamins to non-AIDS patients, however, is fairly well understood.* The importance of several vitamins to the general, non-AIDS patient population is briefly discussed here.

*References 25, 26, 61, 63, 65, 67, 68, 71–73, 75, 76, 153, 205, 308.

Vitamin B₁₂ Deficiency

A vitamin B$_{12}$ deficiency (pernicious anemia) may impair immune function.† In individuals with primary pernicious anemia, the lymphocyte response to mitogens is impaired and neutrophilic, phagocytic, and bactericidal capacity is reduced.[25, 26]

Pyridoxine Deficiency

A pyridoxine (vitamin B$_6$) deficiency results in depressed cellular and humoral immunity in animals. Because of the impairment of DNA and protein synthesis observed in the presence of pyridoxine deficiency, antibody responses to vaccines may be reduced. In addition, delayed cutaneous hypersensitivity reactions are absent and the normal proliferative response of B- and T-lymphocytes does not occur when a pyridoxine deficiency is present.[25, 26]

Pantothenic Acid Deficiency

A pantothenic acid deficiency depresses the antibody response to a primary or booster vaccination by apparently inhibiting the stimulation of antibody-producing cells by antigens.[25, 26]

Vitamin C Deficiency

A vitamin C deficiency impairs cell-mediated immunity.[61, 63, 66–68, 71, 72, 75]

Vitamin A Deficiency

A vitamin A deficiency in animals results in depletion of thymic lymphocytes, depressed lymphocyte response to various mitogens, and increased susceptibility to infections. In humans, secretory IgA production[25, 26] and T-cell function[204] may also be impaired.

Other Vitamin Deficiencies

Thiamine, riboflavin, niacin or biotin deficiencies appear to have little effect, at this time, on immunocompetence.[25, 26]

THERAPEUTIC GOAL

The primary goal of nutritional therapy is to maintain nutritional homeostasis (normal nutritional indices, positive nitrogen balance, and a stable weight). Nutritionists may use the Prognostic Nutritional Index (discussed next) or specific screening criteria to select PWAs who are potential nutritional therapy candidates.

†References 61, 63, 68, 69, 71, 73, 75, 76, 153.

Those who are candidates should undergo a thorough nutritional assessment. They are then treated with a special oral, nasointestinal, enteral, or parenteral diet regimen. Throughout the course of therapy, their therapeutic response is closely monitored by collecting weekly blood samples for testing (serum total protein, albumin, and transferrin levels) and urine (24-hour nitrogen balance) samples.

Prognostic Nutritional Index

Buzby et al.[52] created the Prognostic Nutritional Index (PNI);

$$158 - (A \times 16.6) - (TS \times 0.78) - (T \times 0.2) - (SSF \times 5.8) = \% \text{ risk*}$$

Where A = albumin (g%), TS = triceps skinfold (mm), T = Transferrin (mg%), and SSF = skin sensitivity factor.

This simple equation was designed to determine when preoperative nutrition is indicated in non-AIDS patients. Their studies revealed that preoperative patients with a PNI >40% had an increased risk of postoperative morbidity and mortality. Therefore, they recommended preoperative nutritional therapy for patients with a PNI >40%. This equation may also prove helpful in selecting those PWAs who would most benefit from aggressive nutritional therapy.

Screening Criteria And Nutritional Assessment

At present, there are no well-established nutritional therapy guidelines for malnourished PWAs. Therefore, the author's approach has been to combine specific screening criteria and existing basic nutritional assessment guidelines to evaluate their nutritional status.

Screening Criteria

The screening criteria requires that all PWAs considered for nutritional therapy must first have either (1) an unintentional 10% decrease in their reference weight *or* (2) at least a 20-lb weight loss compared with their usual weight. Patients who satisfy at least one of these criteria undergo a complete physical examination and a nutritional assessment.

*Buzby GP, et al: Prognostic nutritional index in gastrointestinal surgery. *Am J Surg* 1980; 139:160–166. Used by permission.

Nutritional Assessment

The nutritional assessment involves

1. An evaluation of key nutritional indices: protein (visceral and somatic) and fat reserves.
2. A 24-hour nitrogen balance determination.
3. Assessment of gastrointestinal function.
4. An estimate of the patient's daily caloric and protein requirements (see **Chapter 1**).[145]

Visceral protein reserve is estimated from the serum total protein, albumin, and transferrin levels; total lymphocyte count; and antigen skin testing.

Somatic (skeletal) protein reserve is estimated by collecting a 24-hour urine specimen and quantitating the total amount of creatinine (mg) present. This value is then compared to the amount of creatinine (mg) excreted by a well-nourished, non-AIDS (only comparison currently available), stressed individual of the same weight (kg) and height (cm). This comparison is referred to as the creatinine/height index.

Fat reserve is determined per anthropometric measurement of the patient's triceps skinfold. Of all three indices, most nutritionists consider the visceral protein reserve to be the most important index of nutritional status. Table 4–4 lists the normal values for each of these indices and categorizes the values in terms of mild, moderate, and severe malnutrition. Nutritional therapy is indicated when these indices suggest either moderate or severe malnutrition.

A 24-hour nitrogen balance determination is used to evaluate the dynamic relationship between nitrogen utilization and nitrogen loss.[101, 103, 199] Figure 4–7 displays the equation routinely used to calculate a 24-hour nitrogen balance. All PWAs receiving enteral or parenteral nutritional therapy should undergo a weekly 24-hour nitrogen balance determination.

The patients' gastrointestinal function should also be evaluated during the initial nutritional assessment. Those with normal or minimal gut dysfunction may be treated with a low-fat, regular diet supplemented with oral food supplements (see **Normal Gut Function** under **Specific Therapeutic Regimens**). In contrast, PWAs with moderate or severe gut dysfunction require special enteral or parenteral diet therapy or a combination of both (see **Compromised Gut Function** under **Specific Therapeutic Regimens**).

TABLE 4–4.

ARC/AIDS Nutritional Assessment

CLINICAL/LABORATORY PARAMETERS	EXTENT OF MALNUTRITION		
	MILD	MODERATE*	SEVERE*
Albumin, gm/dL†	2.8–3.2	2.1–2.7	<2.1
Transferrin, mg/dL†	150–200	100–150	<100
Total lymphocyte count, cells/mm³†	1,200–2,000	800–1,200	<800
Creatinine/height index (%), actual/ideal × 100‡	60–80	40–60	<40
Ideal body weight, %	80–90	70–80	<70
Usual body weight, %	85–95	75–85	<75
Weight loss/unit time	<5%/mo	<2%/wk	>2%/wk
	<7.5%/3 mo	>5%/mo	
	<10%/6 mo	>7.5%/3 mo	
		>10%/6 mo	
Skin tests			
(No. reactive/no. placed)	4/4	1–2/4	0/0
	(Normal)	(Weak)	(Anergic)

Normal Anthropometric Measurements	MEN	WOMEN
Triceps skinfold, (mm)§	12.5	16.5
Mid-arm circumference (cm)	29.3	28.5

*Nutritional therapy indicated
†Visceral protein reserve
‡Somatic protein reserve
§Fat reserve

A PWA's estimated caloric and protein requirements vary from one clinical situation to another. The caloric requirement for weight maintenance in the general, non-AIDS population ranges from 30 to 35 kcal/kg (usual weight) per day. In the author's experience, however, the daily caloric requirement of PWAs is slightly greater, i.e., 40 to 45 kcal/kg (usual weight) per day to achieve nutritional homeostasis and prevent continued weight loss. A PWA's caloric requirements may be calculated using the equation displayed in Table 4–5 or determined by indirect calorimetry.

The protein requirement for weight maintenance in the general, non-AIDS population ranges from 0.8 to 1.5 g/kg (usual weight) per day. Metabolically stressed patients may require as

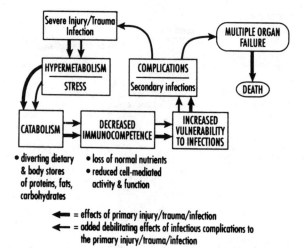

FIG 4–7.
24-Hour nitrogen balance determination.

much as 2.0 to 2.5 g protein/kg (usual weight) per day. The protein requirement of PWAs mimics that of metabolically stressed patients. They should receive 2.0 to 2.5 g/kg (usual weight) to achieve positive nitrogen balance, maintain nutritional homeostasis, and avoid continued weight loss. The diet should deliver 100 to 150 non-protein carbohydrate calories per gram of nitrogen to avoid metabolic and hepatic dysfunction.

Therapeutic Monitoring

A PWA's response to nutritional therapy must be closely monitored. Prior to initiating therapy, a complete nutritional assessment is performed. Then a repeat nutritional assessment, including blood chemistries and a 24-hour nitrogen balance determination, is performed weekly throughout the course of therapy. By monitoring patients in this manner, the author has successfully delivered safe, cost-effective nutrition to several malnourished PWAs.

TABLE 4–5.

Adult ARC/AIDS Daily Caloric and Protein Requirements

Estimate

  Calories (total kcal)

    Male/female: 35–40/kg

  Protein (g)

    Male/female: 2.0–2.5/kg

Calculate

  Calories (total kcal) for weight maintenance

  Male   = $[66.5 + (13.7 \times \text{wt kg}) + (5 \times \text{ht cm}) - (6.7 \times \text{age yr})] \times$ AF*$\times$ IF† + 500 kcal

  Female = $[665.1 + (9.6 \times \text{wt kg}) + (1.8 \times \text{ht cm}) - (4.7 \times \text{age yr})] \times$ AF* $\times$ IF† + 500 kcal

    Note: Add 500 kcal to the equations above for weight gain

  Protein (g)

    Male/female = Total kcal $\times \dfrac{\text{g nitrogen}}{150 \text{ kcal}} \times \dfrac{6.25 \text{ g protein}}{\text{g nitrogen}}$

*Activity factor		†Injury factor	
Confined to bed	1.2	Surgery	1.1–1.2
Ambulatory	1.3	Infection	1.2–1.6
Fever factor	1.13/°C >37°.	Trauma	1.1–1.8
		Sepsis	1.4–1.8.

TREATMENT OPTIONS

General Facts

Several diets have been used to treat malnourished PWAs. They vary in the following ways:

1. Carbohydrate, protein, fat, branched chain amino acid, glutamine, mineral, vitamin, trace metal, pectin, and lactose content.
2. Digestive requirements.
3. Cost.
4. Overall nutritional benefit.

At present, however, no specific oral, enteral or parenteral diet regimen has been shown to be clinically superior.

Most nutritionists agree that the ideal oral or nasointestinal enteral diet for PWAs should

1. Provide low molecular weight (MW) proteins (MW <500 daltons) in the form of either free amino acids or polypeptides.
2. Contain minimal fat (<3% of the total calories) and no lactose.
3. Have a high concentration of branched-chain amino acids (>20% of the total amino acid content) and glutamine (>10% of the total amino acid content).
4. Provide an adequate amount of electrolytes, minerals, and trace metals (selenium, chromium, molybdenum, zinc, copper, iron, and iodine).
5. Contain pectin or have a high-fiber content.
6. Deliver 100 to 150 non-protein carbohydrate calories per gram of nitrogen.
7. Be inexpensive.
8. Provide maximal nutritional benefit.
9. Be consumed either orally or through a small-caliber nasointestinal feeding tube.

The ideal parenteral diet should

1. Deliver maximum caloric ($D_{60}W$) and protein (10% or 15% amino acids) benefit.
2. Provide the required daily electrolytes, minerals, vitamins, and trace metals (selenium, chromium, molybdenum, zinc, copper, iron, and iodine).
3. Contain branched-chain amino acids (>20% of the total amino acid content) and glutamine (>10% of the total amino acid content).
4. Include fat emulsion therapy (5% to 10% of the estimated daily caloric requirement).

Normal Gut Function

In general, PWAs with normal gut function are treated with intact protein, lactose-free, low-fat oral diets. In addition, they are often given Vivonex T.E.N. (free amino acid, elemental), Resource (intact protein), or Carnation Instant Breakfast (intact protein) oral food supplements (see **Types of Diets** and Table 4–6).

Patients with normal gut function who cannot tolerate oral feedings are treated with special enteral diets infused through a nasointestinal feeding tube. The most commonly administered nasointestinal, enteral diets include Vivonex T.E.N., Compleat Modified Formula (intact protein, blenderized, meat-based) or Impact (immuno-enriched). Each of these diets is discussed under **Types of Diets** and in Table 4–6.

Compromised Gut Function

Patients with compromised gut function rarely tolerate intact protein, lactose-free, low-fat oral or enteral diets. Instead, they must be treated with special enteral diets containing protein in the form of low molecular weight, free amino acids or polypeptides. These diets should also:

1. Contain minimal fat (<3% of the total calories) and no lactose.
2. Have a high concentration of branched-chain amino acids (<20% of the total amino acids content) and glutamine (>10% of the total amino acids content).
3. Provide an adequate amount of electrolytes, minerals, vitamins, and trace metals (selenium, chromium, molybdenum, zinc, copper, iron, and iodine).
4. Contain pectin or have a high-fiber content.

Patients with compromised gut function frequently tolerate special diets such as Vivonex T.E.N. Reabilan HN (low molecular weight, polypeptide), Impact, or Compleat Modified Formula when oral diets are not tolerated. These diets must be infused through a nasointestinal feeding tube. Each of these diets is discussed under **Types of Diets** and in Table 4–6.

Patients who fail to tolerate a special, nasointestinal enteral diet are treated with a parenteral diet. Those requiring short-term nutritional therapy (<10 days) may be treated with peripheral parenteral nutrition (PPN); those requiring long-term therapy (>10 days) may be treated with central total parenteral nutrition (TPN). Both parenteral diets are discussed under **Parenteral Diets.**

TYPES OF DIETS

Free Amino Acid, Elemental, Oral And Nasointestinal Enteral Diet

Vivonex T.E.N. (Norwich Eaton Pharmaceuticals, Norwich, New York)[244] is a free amino acid, elemental, oral or nasointestinal enteral diet (see Table 4–6). It has proved to be an excellent oral food supplement or nasointestinal enteral diet for PWAs with either normal or compromised gut function. The diet contains protein in the form of free amino acids. All of the amino acids in

TABLE 4–6.
Composition of Commonly Administered Enteral Diets

Infusion Rate, cc/hr*	1/4			1/2			3/4			Full		
	(40)	(80)	(125)	(40)	(80)	(125)	(40)	(80)	(125)	(40)	(80)	(125)
Vivonex T.E.N.												
NPCC	240	480	744	480	960	1,488	720	1,440	2,232	960	1,920	2,976
P	9	18	28	19	38	59	28	56	87	37	74	115
Reabilan												
NPCC	240	480	744	480	960	1488	720	1440	2,232	960	1,920	2,976
P	8	16	25	15	30	47	23	46	71	30	60	93
Compleat Modified Formula												
NPCC	257	514	797	514	1,028	1,593	770	1,540	2,387	1,027	2,054	3,184
P	10	20	31	21	42	65	31	62	96	41	82	127
Ensure HN												
NPCC	255	510	791	509	1,018	1,578	764	1,528	2,368	1,018	2,036	3,156
P	11	22	34	22	44	68	32	64	99	43	86	133
Nutren 1.0												
NPCC	240	480	744	480	960	1,488	720	1,440	2,232	960	1,920	2,976
P	10	20	31	19	-38	59	29	58	90	38	76	118

Enteral Diet Strength

Isocal												
NPCC	255	510	791	1,018	509	1,578	764	1,528	2,368	1,018	2,036	3,156
P	8	16	25	34	17	53	25	50	78	33	66	102
Osmolite												
NPCC	255	510	791	1,018	509	1,578	764	1,528	2,368	1,018	2,036	3,156
P	9	18	28	36	18	56	27	54	84	36	72	112
Nutren 1.5												
NPCC	360	720	1,116	1,440	720	2,232	1,080	2,160	3,348	1,440	2,880	4,464
P	14	28	43	58	29	90	43	86	133	58	116	180
Nutren 2.0												
NPCC	480	960	1,488	1,920	960	2,976	1,440	2,880	4,464	1,920	3,840	5,952
P	19	38	59	78	39	121	58	116	180	77	154	239
Isocal HCN												
NPCC	480	960	1,488	1,920	960	2,976	1,440	2,880	4,464	1,920	3,840	5,952
P	18	36	56	72	36	112	54	108	167	72	144	223
Pulmocare												
NPCC	360	720	1,116	1,440	720	2,232	1,080	2,160	3,348	1,440	2,880	4,464
P	15	30	47	60	30	93	45	90	140	60	120	186
Travasorb Renal												
NPCC	324	648	1,004	1,296	648	2,009	972	1,944	3,013	1,296	2,592	4,018
P	6	12	19	22	11	34	17	34	53	22	44	68

Continued.

TABLE 4–6 (cont.).

	Enteral Diet Strength											
	1/4			1/2			3/4			Full		
Infusion Rate, cc/hr*	(40)	(80)	(125)	(40)	(80)	(125)	(40)	(80)	(125)	(40)	(80)	(125)
Travasorb Hepatic												
NPCC	264	528	818	528	1,056	1,637	792	1,584	2,455	1,056	2,112	3,274
P	7	14	22	14	28	43	20	40	62	27	54	84
Impact												
NPCC	240	480	944	480	960	1,488	720	1,440	2,232	960	1,920	2,976
P	14	28	43	24	58	90	43	86	133	55	116	180

*The NPCC and P values are based on the indicated concentration and hourly infusion rate administered over 24 hours.

Vivonex T.E.N. have a molecular weight of less than 500 D. Consequently, they are rapidly absorbed in the presence of compromised gut function.

A 1,000-cc serving of Vivonex T.E.N. provides

- 38 g protein (represents 15.3% of the total calories).
- 3 g of fat (represents 2.5% of the total calories).
- 206 g carbohydrate (represents 82.2% of the total calories).

Vivonex T.E.N. has a high concentration of both branched-chain amino acids (33.1% of the total amino acid content)[40] and glutamine (12.8% of the total amino acid content). It

- Delivers 149 non-protein carbohydrate calories per gram of nitrogen.
- Provides 1 kcal/cc.
- Has an osmolality of 630 mOsm/kg of water.
- Requires minimal digestion.

Because it is packaged in powder form, Vivonex T.E.N. is easily mixed with water or a liquid of choice for oral consumption. Because of its low viscosity, it can easily be administered through a small-calibre nasointestinal feeding tube.

Intact Protein, Modular, Oral Diets And Food Supplements

Resource (Sandoz Nutrition Corp., Minneapolis, Minn)[244] is an excellent, inexpensive, intact protein, modular, oral diet or food supplement for PWAs (see Table 4–6). Resource is available in a powdered form, which makes its storage and handling easy. A 1,000-cc serving of Resource (reconstituted in water) provides

- 37.2 g of protein (represents 14% of the total calories).
- 37.2 g of fat (represents 3.5% of the total calories)
- 145 g of carbohydrate (represents 54.5% of the total calories).

Resource

- Delivers 153 non-protein carbohydrate calories per gram of nitrogen.
- Provides 1.06 kcal/cc.

- Is isotonic.
- Contains pectin.

Because of these characteristics, Resource is an excellent oral diet or food supplement for PWAs with normal or mild gut dysfunction. Resource (1) contains intact protein instead of low molecular weight amino acids or polypeptides; (2) has a relatively high fat content; and (3) lacks branched-chain amino acids, glutamine, and important trace metals (selenium, chromium and molybdenum); therefore, it is not tolerated well by PWAs with moderate or severe gut dysfunction.

Carnation Instant Breakfast by (Baxter Health Care Corp., Deerfield, Ill)[244] is an inexpensive, intact protein, oral diet and food supplement used to treat PWAs with normal or mild gut dysfunction (see Table 4–6). Because Carnation Instant Breakfast is packaged in powdered form, it is simple to store and convenient to use. An unconstituted 1.23-oz envelope of vanilla-flavored Carnation Instant Breakfast

- Provides 7 g protein (15% of the total calories).
- Has less than 1 g fat and 24 g carbohydrate (84% of the total calories).
- Delivers 130 kcal.
- Has a ratio of non-protein carbohydrate to gram of nitrogen of 92:1.
- Contains most of the essential vitamins and minerals and a few of the key trace metals.

Because it contains intact protein and lactose, Carnation Instant Breakfast is poorly tolerated by PWAs with moderate or severe gut dysfunction.

Blenderized, Meat-Based, Intact Protein, Nasointestinal Enteral Diet

Compleat Modified Formula (Sandoz Nutrition Corp., Minneapolis, Minn)[244] is a blenderized, meat-based, intact protein, nasointestinal enteral diet (see Table 4–6). A 1,000-cc serving of Compleat Modified Formula provides

- 43 g protein (represents 16% of the total calories).
- 37 g of fat (30% of the total calories).
- 140 g of carbohydrate (54% of the total calories).

It

- Delivers 131 non-protein carbohydrate calories per gram nitrogen.
- Provides 1.07 kcal/cc.
- Is isotonic.
- Contains pectin.

Because Compleat Modified Formula is isotonic and contains blenderized meat, vegetables, and pectin, it is well tolerated by PWAs with minimal or moderate gut dysfunction. Since Compleat Modified Formula contains intact protein instead of low molecular weight free amino acids or polypeptides and has a relatively high fat content, it is not tolerated well by PWAs with moderate or severe gut dysfunction.

Immuno-Enriched, Intact Protein, Nasointestinal Enteral Diet

Impact (Sandoz Nutrition Corporation, Minneapolis, Minn)[244] is a unique, ready-to-use, immuno-enriched, intact protein, nasointestinal enteral diet (see Table 4–6). A 1,500-cc serving provides

- 84 g of protein (22% of the total calories).
- 42 g of fat (25% of the total calories).
- 198 g of carbohydrate (53% of the total calories).

It

- Delivers 71 non-protein carbohydrate calories per gram of nitrogen.
- Provides 1.0 kcal/cc.
- Has an osmolality of 375 mOsm/kg water.
- Contains the essential vitamins, minerals, and trace metals (selenium, chromium, and molybdenum).

Impact has been specially formulated to provide nutritional support for the immune system under metabolic stress resulting from trauma, sepsis, cancer, burns, or surgery.

Impact contains

1. Arginine, which strongly stimulates lymphocyte reactivity in healthy humans.[20, 92, 265, 325]

2. Additional RNA, which is vital for monitoring normal cellular immunity and host resistance.[111, 187, 320, 321]

3. Additional omega-3 fatty acids and decreased omega-6 fatty acids, which are beneficial in improving the survival of patients at risk for infection.

4. Structured lipids composed of medium-chain triglycerides and long-chain triglycerides, which provide essential fatty acids in a form that is rapidly transported and utilized.[20, 92]

As yet, no clinical studies have been conducted to evaluate the use of Impact in the nutritional management of PWAs. Because of its unique formulation, however, the author believes that Impact may prove to be a beneficial diet for PWAs with normal or mild gut dysfunction.

Low Molecular Weight, Polypeptide, Nasointestinal Enteral Diet

Reabilan HN (O'Brien Pharmaceuticals, Parsippany, NJ),[244] is a low molecular weight, polypeptide, nasointestinal enteral diet (see Table 4–6). A 1,000-cc serving of Reabilan HN provides

- 58 g of protein (17.5% of the total calories).
- 52 g of fat (35% of the total calories).
- 158 g of carbohydrate (48% of the total calories).

It

- Delivers 125 non-protein carbohydrate calories per gram of nitrogen.
- Provides 1.33 kcal/cc.
- Has an osmolality of 490 mOsm/kg of water.
- Contains essential amino acids (43% of the total amino acid content), branched chain amino acids (21% of the total amino acid content), glutamic acid, and the important trace metals (selenium, chromium, and molybdenum).

The most important characteristics of Reabilan HN is its high percentage of low molecular weight polypeptides. Fifty-six percent of the polypeptides in Reabilan HN have MWs less than 1,000 d.

Silk et al.[283] demonstrated that low-MW polypeptides (MW <500 d) were absorbed much faster than amino acids by the intestine. Conversely, they discovered that large polypeptides (MW >500 d) were not absorbed as fast as amino acids. Several other investigators have suggested that diet's content of low-MW poly-peptides (MW <1,000 D) may influence its intestinal absorption.[43–46, 106, 107, 144, 154, 172]

In view of the absorptive characteristics of low-MW polypep-tides (MW <500 d), several nutritionists have attempted to treat PWAs with moderate or severe gut dysfunction with polypeptide diets. Unfortunately, most commercially available polypeptide di-ets do not contain low-MW (MW <500 d) polypeptides. Instead, they usually contain 40% to 80% large polypeptides (MW >1,000 d), which are not absorbed as well as amino acids in the presence of compromised gut function. In addition, polypeptide diets often contain intact protein and have high fat contents, which further compromise their absorption in PWAs with gut dysfunction. Since Reabilan HN, in comparison to other polypeptide diets, has the highest percentage of low-MW polypeptides (MW <1,000 d), it is the author's preferred polypeptide diet. Because Reabilan HN contains 44% large MW polypeptides (MW >1,000 d), however, the author still prefers to treat PWAs with moderate or severe gut dysfunction with a free amino acid, elemental diet.

BRAT Diet

Nutritionists have discovered that the combined administration of a BRAT (bananas, rice, apples, tea or toast) and peripheral par-enteral diet provide an excellent, short-term (<7 days) method for treating PWAs with moderate to severe gut dysfunction and diar-rhea. Unfortunately, the caloric and protein benefits of this nutri-tional regimen are limited. In addition, PWAs are rarely able to tolerate a BRAT diet for an extended period of time because of taste fatigue.

As an alternative to the BRAT diet, many nutritionists are now administering various World Health Organization diets to PWAs with moderate or severe gut dysfunction and diarrhea.[222] Many of these diets have been very effective in reducing the vol-ume and frequency of diarrhea, maintaining hydration, and pro-viding maintenance nutrition.

Parenteral Diets

Parenteral diets provide the most effective nutritional therapy for PWAs. There are basically two methods of parenteral diet therapy: (1) peripheral parenteral nutrition (PPN) therapy (see Ta-bles 3–1, 3–13, and 3–14 for more details) *and* (2) total paren-teral nutrition (TPN) therapy (see Tables 3–1, 3–2, and 3–4 and

Tables 4–7 and 4–8 for more details). Both PPN and TPN therapy are very effective in restoring nutritional homeostasis in malnourished PWAs.[8] Unfortunately, these treatment modalities are very expensive. Because of the cost, the author has established specific criteria for initiating parenteral diet therapy.

Peripheral Parenteral Nutrition

This is utilized as a short-term (<10 days) method of nutritional therapy for neurologically intact,* non-terminal, malnourished PWAs who (1) are unable to successfully consume their required daily caloric and protein requirements via oral or enteral feedings *or* (2) require parenteral diet therapy because they suffer from enteral diet–induced or infectious diarrhea. In general, most nutritionists consider PPN therapy as a temporary, suboptimal method of nutritional therapy in comparison to central TPN. A standard "mixed" PPN solution contains dextrose, amino acids, electrolytes, vitamins, minerals, and trace metals. One liter of PPN solution contains $D_{20}W$, 500 cc, and 10% amino acids (protein), 500 cc. It provides approximately 400 kcal and 50 g of protein or 8 g of nitrogen (1 g of nitrogen = 6.25 g protein). Since a standard PPN solution delivers adequate nitrogen but inadequate calories, PPN therapy must include the daily intravenous infusion of 20% fat emulsion (2 kcal/cc), 500 cc. The continuous infusion of the PPN solution at 125 cc/hour plus the daily administration of 20% fat emulsion, 500 cc, provides approximately 2,200 kcal and 150 g protein. Because PPN therapy provides only maintenance calories and protein, it is considered only when short-term (<10 days) nutritional therapy is required. Tables 3–1, 3–13, and 3–14 discuss the formulation and administration of PPN therapy.

ProcalAmine (McGaw Laboratories, Inc.®, Irvine, Calif)[244] is a unique "pre-mixed" PPN solution which utilizes glycerol, a three-carbon polyalcohol, as its primary caloric source. Studies have shown that glycerol is

1. Gluconeogenic and inhibits gluconeogenesis from amino acids.
2. Insulinogenic to a small degree.
3. Anti-ketogenic.
4. Chemically compatible with amino acids.
5. More calorically dense than glucose.

Because of these physiologic and biochemical properties, glycerol can be combined with amino acids and electrolytes into the same

*References 168, 207, 230, 275, 276, 287, 307, 337.

intravenous solution for protein-sparing therapy. Furthermore, glycerol can serve as an energy substrate for intravenous application in patients who cannot utilize glucose due to specific disease states.*

One liter of ProcalAmine provides

- Glycerol, 30 g (245 kcal).
- Amino acids, 290 g (4.6 g of nitrogen).
- Electrolytes (sodium 35 mEq, potassium 24 mEq, and chloride 41 mEq).
- Minerals (calcium 3 mEq and phosphate 3.5 mM).
- Magnesium 5 mEq.
- Acetate (inorganic salts, 23 mEq; acetic acid, 9 mEq; and lysine acetate, 15 mEq).

ProcalAmine may be utilized as

1. An alternative to dextrose or saline intravenous therapy.
2. A supplement to inadequate oral enteral diet therapy.
3. Short-term (<10 days) maintenance nutritional therapy for patients with gut dysfunction.

ProcalAmine provides an economical, convenient method of maintenance nutritional therapy. Since it is "pre-mixed," the administration of ProcalAmine significantly reduces the formulation time of the physician and the mixing time of the pharmacist. In addition, its usage virtually eliminates the solution wastage associated with the administration of individualized, "mixed" PPN solutions.

Although not as nutritionally beneficial as a "mixed" PPN solution, ProcalAmine is a satisfactory therapeutic alternative for medical facilities with limited pharmaceutical staffing, marginal medical expertise in parenteral diet therapy, or a restricted budget. In view of the geographic distribution of AIDS patients, the escalating cost of AIDS therapy, and the predicted AIDS epidemic, ProcalAmine may provide an effective alternative to "mixed" PPN therapy for PWAs.

Total Parenteral Nutrition

TPN therapy is utilized as a method of long-term (>10 days, <3 months) nutritional therapy for neurologically intact,* nonterminal, malnourished PWAs who are unable to consume their

---

*References 85, 108, 123, 150, 254, 277, 309, 326, 339.

*References 168, 207, 230, 275, 276, 287, 307, 337.

required daily nutrients by oral or enteral feedings while undergoing chemotherapy and antidiarrheal therapy for an enteric infection. If the enteric infection and diarrhea are unsuccessfully treated in 3 months, the TPN therapy should be discontinued. The administration of long-term (>3 months) TPN therapy for intractable diarrhea or enteral diet intolerance is ethically and economically very controversial.*

In the past, antidiarrheal agents, such as Lomotil, Imodium, and deodorized tincture of opium (DTO), were relatively ineffective in treating the diarrhea caused by enteric infections such as *Mycobacterium avium-intracellulare, Salmonella, Campylobacter, Candida albicans, Cryptosporidium, Isospora belli, Microsporidia,* cytomegalovirus, and Herpes simplex virus. Recently, however, the author and several other investigators have successfully used Sandostatin (Sandoz Pharmaceuticals Corp., East Hanover, NJ)[244] to treat the diarrhea caused by several of these infections.

Sandostatin is a synthetic octapeptide with pharmacologic actions mimicking those of the natural hormone somatostatin.[128, 142] Sandostatin has the ability to suppress the secretion of serotonin,[170, 189, 203, 236, 270, 323] vasoactive intestinal polypeptide,[29, 41, 78, 179] gastrin,[10, 130, 278, 304, 324, 341] insulin,[104, 239, 322] glucagon,[6, 10, 36, 209] growth hormone, secretin, and pancreatic polypeptides.[60, 116, 189, 324, 341] It also exerts widespread effects on gastrointestinal function.[126, 234, 324] It prolongs intestinal transit time, regulates intestinal water and electrolyte transport, and decreases splanchnic blood flow.†

Sandostatin differs from native somatostatin in four significant ways: Sandostatin

1. Has a half-life of 60 to 112 minutes with a duration of action of 6 to 12 hours (somatostatin has a half-life of only 1 to 2 minutes).
2. Can be administered subcutaneously or intravenously.
3. Inhibits growth hormone secretion preferentially to insulin secretion.
4. Is associated with less rebound hypersecretion when its affect tapers off.[170, 171]

Diarrhea can be a life-threatening complication of AIDS. As many as 50% to 90% of all AIDS patients have gastrointestinal

---

*References 34, 48, 53, 91, 159, 181, 200, 250, 271, 282, 302, 303, 328, 330.

†References 83, 93, 97, 112, 164, 186, 223, 234, 255, 256.

symptoms during the course of their disease. Diarrhea, usually chronic in nature and associated with weight loss and malnutrition, is the most common symptom.

The exact mechanism for the success of Sandostatin in the treatment of AIDS diarrhea is not well understood. Cook et al.[82] believe that the direct action of Sandostatin on the secretory apparatus of the gut controlled their patients' diarrhea. They also stated that this affect appeared to be mediated by the drug's suppressive action on intestinal transport rather than an affect on immunity. Because the AIDS virus is homologous to a vasoactive intestinal polypeptide (VIP) in its protein code amino acid sequences, Cook et al. have theorized that the AIDS virus may activate VIP receptors that induce the diarrheal response. Since Sandostatin is effective in controlling the secretory diarrhea associated with both AIDS and VIP-secreting tumors, it may be working at a membrane receptor that recognizes the VIP.

The majority of PWAs with diarrhea who responded to Sandostatin therapy in the literature were infected with the coccidioidal protozoan *Cryptosporidium*. This pathogen inhibits the microvillus border of the intestinal epithelial cells and is a common cause for severe, secretory diarrhea in immunosuppressed PWAs. The clinical manifestations of this cryptosporidial infection include severe watery diarrhea, abdominal cramping, malabsorption, and weight loss. Since the diarrhea is refractory to conventional antidiarrheal therapy (e.g., deodorized tincture of opium (DTO), Lomotil, and Imodium), patients frequently require hospitalization, intravenous fluids, and electrolyte replacement.

At present, most case reports indicate that Sandostatin can be successfully utilized to significantly reduce the volume of diarrhea in 30% to 40% of PWAs with *Cryptosporidium*-induced secretory diarrhea.

Rene et al.[252] reported a significant reduction of stool output in two AIDS patients with isolated cryptosporidiosis following the subcutaneous administration of Sandostatin 100 μg twice daily.

Robinson and Fuegel[256] presented a case involving a man with AIDS-associated diarrhea without a demonstrable cryptosporidial infection. Sandostatin therapy was initiated at a dosage of 50 μg twice daily and eventually increased to three times daily. The patient's diarrhea rapidly ceased, his appetite improved, and he gained 9 kg in 6 weeks. Following 10 weeks of treatment, he had maintained his weight and experienced no further problems with diarrhea.

Fuessl et al.[125-127] used Sandostatin to treat two PWAs who had "uncontrollable diarrhea." The diarrhea was attributed to cytomegalovirus (CMV) enteritis. In these patients, Sandostatin therapy resulted in prompt improvement in both the frequency and volume of stools.

Further studies are clearly necessary to determine the role and mechanism of action of Sandostatin in the treatment of AIDS-related diarrhea. The preliminary reports from several ongoing clinical trials evaluating the effectiveness of Sandostatin in controlling AIDS diarrhea are very encouraging.[82, 171, 218, 256, 257, 286] In view of this, the author now believes that short-term (>10 days, <3 months) combined TPN and Sandostatin therapy should be administered to PWAs who have satisfied *all* of the following treatment criteria:

1. A recent 10% decrease in usual weight or a 20-lb weight loss.
2. Abnormal nutritional indices.
3. A *Cryptosporidium* or cytomegalovirus intestinal infection causing massive diarrhea (>800 cc/day) that is refractory to chemotherapy and antidiarrheal therapy.
4. An intolerance of both oral and nasointestinal enteral diet therapy.
5. No central nervous system disease.
6. The emotional stability to cope with prolonged parenteral diet therapy.
7. The intellectual capacity and technical skill to safely self-administer a parenteral diet.
8. A social and living environment which supports long-term parenteral diet therapy.
9. Agreed to accept the treating physician's recommendations regarding the duration and termination of parenteral diet therapy.

A liter of TPN solution for PWAs should contain $D_{60}W$, 500 cc, and 10% amino acids (protein), 500 cc plus routine and optional additives. It provides approximately 1,200 kcal and 50 g of protein or 8 g of nitrogen (1 g of nitrogen = 6.25 g protein). The solution has a ratio of non-protein carbohydrate calories to grams nitrogen of 150:1 (1,200 kcal ÷ 8 g of nitrogen = 150). The solution is initially infused at a rate of 40 cc/hour. A final infusion rate of 100 to 125 cc/hour should be achieved within 48 to 72 hours. The final infusion rate is dependent on the PWA's esti-

TABLE 4–7.
Basic Formulation of 1 L of Standard ARC/AIDS TPN Therapy

COMPONENTS	
Routine additives	**Dosage**
$D_{60}W^*$	500 cc
10% Amino acid*	500 cc
Sodium chloride†	0–130 mEq
Sodium phosphate‡	0–20 mM
Potassium chloride§	0–40 mEq
Magnesium sulfate¶	8–12 mEq
Ca gluconate¶,‖	4.5 or 9.0 mEq
MVI-12**	10cc
Multitrace**	5cc
Optional additives	**Dosage**
Sodium Acetate†	0–130 mEq
Potassium Acetate§	0–40 mEq
H_2 Antagonist††	
Albumin (25%)‡‡	25 g
Regular Insulin§§	0–40 units

ADMINISTRATION SCHEDULE	
Day of Therapy	**Rate (cc/hr)**
1	40
2	80
3	100–125¶¶

FAT EMULSION INFUSION SCHEDULE

Infuse a 20% fat emulsion 500 cc intravenously per pump over 6–8 hr at least 3 times per week via either an 18-gauge peripheral intravenous cannula or piggyback per the central infusion catheter.

---

*The solution should be formulated to deliver 100–150 non-protein carbohydrate calories per gram of nitrogen infused.
†Add sodium chloride if the serum CO_2 >25 mEq/L. Add sodium acetate if the serum CO_2 ≤25 mEq/L.
‡The total phosphate dosage should not exceed 20 mM/L or 60 mM daily.
§Add KCl if the serum CO_2 >25mEq/L. Add K acetate if the serum CO_2 ≤25 mEq/L. The potassium dosage should not exceed 40mEq per liter.
¶Added to each liter.
‖Add calcium gluceptate 9 mEq to each liter if the serum calcium <8.5mEq/L. Add 4.5 mEq if the serum calcium ≥8.5mEq/L.
**Administered in only 1 L/day.
††Dosage variable. Consult the *Physicians' Desk Reference* and add an equal dose to each liter.
‡‡25% albumin 25 g is added to each liter if the serum albumin <2.5gm% and enteral diet therapy is anticipated.
§§Total dosage should not exceed 40 units per liter.
¶¶The final infusion rate is dependent upon the patient's calculated daily caloric and protein requirements and overall cardiovascular status.

TABLE 4–8.

ARC/AIDS Central TPN Therapy Orders

TPN 1. Components	Recommended Dosage Ranges per Liter TPN	Bag No. ___	Bag No. ___	Bag No. ___
Routine Additives				
$D_{60}W$	500 cc	500 cc	500 cc	500 cc
10% AA	500 cc	500 cc	500 cc	500 cc
NaCl	0–140 mEq	mEq	mEq	mEq
NaPO4	0–20 mM	mM	mM	mM
KCl*	0–40 mEq	mEq	mEq	mEq
$MgSO_4$	8–12 mEq	mEq	mEq	mEq
Ca gluconate	4.5 or 9 mEq	mEq	mEq	mEq
MVI-12	10 cc/day	10 cc		
Multitrace	5 cc/day	5 cc		
Optional Additives				
Na acetate	0–140 mEq	mEq	mEq	mEq
K* acetate	0–40 mEq	mEq	mEq	mEq
Regular insulin	0–40 units	units	units	units
H_2 antagonist†	—	—	—	—
25% albumin‡	25 gm	gm	gm	gm
Nurse's signature				

RATE: __40__ cc/hr via pump.

Final dextrose concentration __30__ % Final AA concentration __5__ %

2. Pharmacy to add vitamin K 10 mg to 1 L of TPN q Mon. and Thurs.
3. Fat emulsion 20% 500 cc q Mon., Wed. and Fri. IVPB per pump over 6–8 hr via at least an 18-gauge peripheral IV or the subclavian catheter.
4. STAT upright and expirational portable CXR to check the position of the subclavian catheter and to R/O a pneumothorax. Notify the physician when the CXR is completed.
5. Heparin lock the TPN catheter with 2 cc of heparin (100 units/cc) until notified by the physician to start the first liter of TPN.
6. Strict I/O q shift. Total the I/O q 24 hr.
7. Record the daily weight in kg on the vital signs sheet.
8. Check the urine for sugar and acetone q shift and record on the vital signs sheet. If the urine sugar is **4+**, request a STAT serum glucose to be drawn by the physician. If the serum glucose >**160 mg%**, contact the physician for treatment orders.
9. Notify the physician if the oral temperature >**38° C**.
10. Routine TPN labs are to be drawn weekly on the days and the times specified below:
    Sun. A.M.: CBC, SMAC-20
    Tues. A.M.: Electrolytes, BUN, creatinine, and glucose
    Thurs. A.M.: CBC, SMAC-20, copper, zinc, magnesium, transferrin, triglyceride, pre-albumin, and retinol binding protein
11. Begin a 24-hour urine collection for urinary urea nitrogen (UUN) at 6:00 A.M. q Mon. and Thurs. for nitrogen balance determination.
12. TPN catheter dressing and tubing changes per the hospital TPN protocol.
13. Contact the physician for all problems related to TPN.
14. All changes in TPN therapy must be approved by the physician.

*Total potassium content per liter of TPN should not exceed 40mEq.
†Divide the daily dosage equally into each liter of TPN.
‡Only if the serum albumin <2.5gm% and enteral diet therapy is anticipated.

mated daily caloric and protein requirements, age, and overall cardiovascular status.

Patients treated with TPN therapy should also receive at least 4% to 6% of their daily caloric requirement as fat. This is accomplished by routinely administering 20% fat emulsion (2 kcal/cc), 500 cc, three times per week. The actual frequency and quantity of fat administered may be increased depending on the patient's caloric requirements, clinical situation, or pulmonary function. Fat therapy should not, however, provide more than 50% of a PWA's estimated daily caloric requirement.* Tables 3–1, 3–2, and 3–4 and Tables 4–7 and 4–8 discuss the basic formulation and administration of TPN therapy.

SPECIFIC THERAPEUTIC REGIMENS

Prior to receiving nutritional therapy, PWAs must satisfy the therapeutic screening criteria previously discussed (see **Screening Criteria and Nutritional Assessment**). In addition, they must be separated into two groups based on gut function. PWAs with normal gut function are treated according to the algorithm discussed subsequently under **Normal Gut Function** or summarized in Table 4–9. Patients with compromised gut function are thoroughly evaluated and then grouped based on their type of enteropathy: "nonspecific," "enteropathic," "colitic," and "cholerrheic."[184] Then, depending on the enteropathy present, a specific nutritional therapy algorithm is followed. The different enteropathies and their treatment algorithms are discussed under **Compromised Gut Function** or summarized in Table 4–9.

Normal Gut Function

Oral Diet

Patients with normal gut function who can tolerate oral feedings should be treated with a high-calorie, high-protein, low-fat (<3% of the total daily caloric intake), lactose-free, oral diet. The diet should be carefully designed based on the patient's food preferences and nutritional requirements. In addition to the diet, they should receive Vivonex T.E.N. oral food supplements. If the patient is unable to tolerate the Vivonex T.E.N., then either Resource or Carnation Instant Breakfast oral food supplements may be substituted.

*References 136, 193, 198, 201, 205, 206, 288.

TABLE 4–9.
ARC/AIDS Nutritional Therapy Algorithms

NORMAL GUT FUNCTION	COMPROMISED GUT FUNCTION	
	Nonspecific and Enteropathic Enteropathy	Colitic and Cholerrheic Enteropathy
STEP 1	**STEP 1**	**STEP 1**
Oral diet	**Oral diet**	**Nasointestinal enteral diet**
High-caloric, high-protein, low-fat (<3% total daily caloric intake), lactose-free	High-caloric, high-protein low-fat (<3% total daily caloric intake), lactose-free	Vivonex T.E.N., full-strength, nasointestinal enteral diet continuously at 100–125 cc/hr per volumetric pump
plus	**plus**	**or**
Oral food supplements	**Oral food supplements**	Peptamen, full-strength, nasointestinal enteral diet continuously at 100–125 cc/hr per volumetric pump
Vivonex T.E.N., 4–8 packets reconstituted, full-strength in chilled water, juice or soft drink	Vivonex T.E.N., 4–8 packets reconstituted, full-strength in chilled water, juice, or soft drink	**or**
or	**or**	Impact, full-strength continuously at 100–125 cc/hr per volumetric pump
Resource, 4–8 packets reconstituted, full-strength in water	Resource, 4–8 packets reconstituted, full-strength in water	**or**
or	**or**	Compleat Modified Formula, full-strength, nasointestinal enteral diet continuously at 100–125 cc/hr per volumetric pump
Carnation Instant Breakfast, 4–6 packets reconstituted, full-strength in vitamin D whole milk	Carnation Instant Breakfast, 4–6 packets reconstituted, full-strength in vitamin D whole milk	

STEP 2
Nasointestinal enteral diet
Vivonex T.E.N., full-strength, continuously at 100–125 cc/hr per volumetric pump

or

Compleat Modified Formula, full-strength, continuously at 100–125 cc/hr per volumetric pump

or

Impact, full-strength, continuously at 100–125 cc/hr per volumetric pump

or

Peptamen, full-strength, continuously at 100–125 cc/hr per volumetric pump

plus

Antidiarrheal agents (descending order of preference):
Sandostatin 50–300 µg SQ or IV q 6 hr prn

or

Lomotil 1–2 tabs (2.5 mg/tab) po q 6 hr prn

or

Imodium 1–2 caps (2 mg/cap) po q 6 hr prn

or

Deodorized tincture of opium (DTO) 15–20 gtt po q 4–6 hr prn

or

STEP 2
Nasointestinal enteral diet
Vivonex T.E.N. full-strength, nasointestinal enteral diet continuously at 100–125 cc/hr per volumetric pump

or

Compleat Modified Formula, full-strength, nasointestinal enteral diet continuously at 100–125 cc/hr per volumetric pump

(Continued.)

plus

Antidiarrheal agents (descending order of preference):
Sandostatin 50–300 uqm SQ or IV q 6 hr prn

or

Lomotil 1–2 tabs (2.5 mg/tab) po q 6 hr prn

or

Imodium 1–2 caps (2 mg/cap) po q 6 hr prn

or

Deodorized tincture of opium (DTO) 15–20 gtt po q 4–6 hr prm

plus

STEP 2
Peripheral parenteral nutrition (PPN)
"Mixed" continuously, at 125 cc/hr per volumetric pump for <10 days

or

"Premixed" ProcalAmine continuously at 125 cc/hr per volumetric pump for <10 days

(Continued.)

TABLE 4–9 (cont.).
ARC/AIDS Nutritional Therapy Algorithms

	COMPROMISED GUT FUNCTION	
	Nonspecific and Enteropathic Enteropathy	Colitic and Cholerrheic Enteropathy
	or	*plus*
	Impact, full-strength, continuously at 100–125 cc/hr per volumetric pump	Fat emulsion, 20% 500 cc intravenously over 4–6 hr daily
	or	*plus*
	Peptamen, full-strength, continuously at 100–l25 cc/hr per volumetric pump	***STEP 3***
	plus	Antidiarrheal agents (same as in Step 1 above)
	Antidiarrheal agents (descending order of preference):	Total parenteral nutrition (TPN) continuously at 100–125 cc/hr per volumetric pump (>10 days <3 months)
	Sandostatin 50–300 μg SQ or IV q 6 hr prm	*plus*
	Lomotil 5–10 cc (2.5 mg/cc) via the nasointestinal feeding tube q 4–6 hr prm	Fat emulsion 20% 500 cc intravenously over 4–6 hr at least 3 times per week
	or	*plus*
	Imodium 10–20 cc (1 mg/cc) via the nasointestinal feeding tube q 6 hr prm	Antidiarrheal agents (same as Step 1)
	or	
	Deodorized tincture of opium (DTO) 15–20 gtt via the nasointestinal feeding tube q 4–6 hr prm	

or

STEP 3

Peripheral parenteral nutrition (PPN)

"Mixed" continuously at 125 cc/hr per volumetric pump for <10 days

or

"Premixed" ProcalAmine continuously at 125 cc/hr per volumetric pump for <10 days

plus

Fat emulsion 20% 500 cc intravenously over 4–6 hr daily

plus

Antidiarrheal agents (same as in Step 1 above)

STEP 4

Total parenteral nutrition (TPN)

continuously at 100–125 cc/hr per volumetric pump (>10 days <3 months)

plus

Fat emulsion 20% 500 cc intravenously over 4–6 hr 3 times per week

plus

Antidiarrheal agents (same as in Step 1 above)

Patients with AIDS often take appetite stimulants to increase their oral food consumption.[210, 211] These stimulants have had variable success. Recently, many PWAs have used Megace (Bristol-Myers, New York, NY)[244] as an appetite stimulant. Megace is an antineoplastic agent approved by the Federal Drug Administration for the treatment of breast and endometrial carcinoma. At present, it has not been approved as an appetite stimulant. Because of this, the author does not recommend Megace as an appetite stimulant.

Nasointestinal Enteral Diet

PWAs with normal gut function who are unable to tolerate oral feedings are treated with a nasointestinal enteral diet. The author has successfully treated several PWAs with Vivonex T.E.N. administered through a nasointestinal feeding tube. Other nutritionists have reported variable success with Impact, Reabilan HN, and Compleat Modified Formula. Although nasointestinal feedings are easy to administer, patients rarely tolerate them for an extended period of time. They usually begin to complain of a sore throat, auditory deficits, or nasal congestion. Because of these complaints, the nutritionist is forced to use an alternative method of nutritional therapy, such as oral or parenteral diet therapy.

In addition to the diet therapy discussed here, patients should also receive daily vitamin, mineral, and trace metal supplements either orally or in their nasointestinal feeding tube.

Compromised Gut Function

Patients with AIDS often have compromised gut function. Kotler has described and classified the different enteropathies which occur in PWAs.[181, 185] He has grouped the gut dysfunction into four specific types of enteropathies: "non-specific," "enteropathic," "colitic," and "cholerrheic." The different types of enteropathies are defined according to

1. The portion of the gut involved.
2. The frequency of bowel movements and the texture of the stool produced.
3. The patient's associated gastrointestinal complaints and appetite.
4. The degree of electrolyte deficiencies and dehydration.
5. Extent of malabsorption and weight loss.
6. Intolerance to lactose and fat.
7. The bacteriologic etiology for the diarrhea.

The author has carefully designed specific nutritional therapy algorithms for each of these enteropathies (see Table 4–9).

Diet for Nonspecific Enteropathy

Malnourished PWAs who have a good appetite, minimal gut dysfunction, modest gastrointestinal symptoms, and semisolid stool (i.e., "nonspecific enteropathy") are treated according to the following algorithm. Initially, they are treated with a special high-calorie, high-protein, low-fat (<3% total daily caloric intake), lactose-free, oral diet plus 4 to 8 packets of Vivonex T.E.N. (reconstituted full-strength in chilled water, juice or soft drink) oral food supplements. If the patient is unable to tolerate the Vivonex T.E.N.®, then 4 to 8 packets of Resource (reconstituted full-strength in water) or Carnation Instant Breakfast 4–6 packets (reconstituted full-strength in vitamin D whole milk) may be substituted. The food supplement dosage is dependent upon the patient's oral diet consumption and estimated daily caloric and protein requirement (see Table 4–5).

Patients who develop diarrhea as a result of this therapy should continue with their oral diet and food supplements but also receive antidiarrheal therapy. The most effective antidiarrheal agents (in descending order of preference) include:

1. Sandostatin, 50 to 300 µg subcutaneously every 6 hours prn.[245]
2. Imodium, 1 to 2 capsules (2 mg/cap) orally every 6 hours prn.
3. Deodorized tincture of opium (DTO), 15 to 20 drops orally every 4 to 6 hours prn.
4. Lomotil, 1 to 2 tablets (2.5 mg/tab) orally every 4 to 6 hours prn.

PWAs who are unable to tolerate an oral diet but can tolerate Vivonex T.E.N. are treated with Vivonex T.E.N. administered via a nasointestinal feeding tube. The Vivonex T.E.N. is infused according to the hyperosmolar infusion schedule displayed in Table 4–10.

Patients unable to tolerate the Vivonex T.E.N. nasointestinal enteral diet (persistent or increased diarrhea) may be treated with Impact or Reabilan HN enteral diets. If the patient is unable to tolerate these diets, then Compleat Modified Formula enteral diet should be administered. The Compleat Modified Formula is infused per the isosmolar infusion schedule displayed in Table 4–10. In addition, these patients should receive antidiarrheal therapy through the nasointestinal feeding tube or subcutaneously (see Table 4–9).

Patients unable to tolerate the Compleat Modified Formula nasointestinal enteral diet (persistent or diarrhea) are treated with a short course (<10 days) peripheral parenteral nutrition (PPN), bowel rest, and antidiarrheal therapy. Patients who respond to this treatment regimen and whose gut function returns to normal are restarted on either an oral or one of the nasointestinal enteral diets previously discussed.

Patients who fail a short course of PPN therapy (i.e., gut function fails to return to normal) may be considered for long-term (>10 days, <3 months) central TPN therapy. These patients, however, must satisfy the selection criteria previously discussed.

In addition to these various diet regimens, PWAs with a "nonspecific" enteropathy should also receive daily vitamin, mineral and trace metal supplements. Table 4–9 summarizes the nutritional therapy algorithm for a "nonspecific enteropathy."

Diet for Enteropathic Enteropathy

Malnourished PWAs who have moderate frequency, watery diarrhea associated with electrolyte deficiencies and malabsorption (i.e., "enteropathic" enteropathy) are treated according to the same nutritional therapy algorithm as PWAs with a "nonspecific" enteropathy (see Table 4–9).

TABLE 4–10.
Enteral Diet Infusion Schedules

Isosmolar			Hyperosmolar		
(280–300 mOsm/kg of H_2O)			(>300 mOsm/kg of H_2O)		
Hr	Strength	Rate (cc/hr via pump)	Hr	Strength	Rate (cc/hr via pump)
12	Full	40	12	1/4	40
12	Full	80	12	1/2	40
12	Full	100–125*	18	3/4	40
			12	Full	40
			12	Full	80
			24	Full	100–125*

*The final infusion rate is dependent on the patient's calculated total caloric and protein requirements, overall cardiovascular status, and tolerance of the diet

Diet for Colitic Enteropathy

The nutritional management of PWAs with massive diarrhea associated with tenesmus, severe cramping, and anorexia (i.e., "colitic" enteropathy) is very challenging. These patients are usually dehydrated, have significant electrolyte abnormalities, respond poorly to antidiarrheal agents, and are severely malnourished.

Because they are severely malnourished, patients with a "colitic" enteropathy often have a serum albumin less than 2.5 g/dL. Hypoalbuminemia adversely effects gut function by lowering the serum colloid osmotic pressure (COP) and bowel wall oncotic pressure (BWOP). The reduced serum COP and BWOP in turn causes impaired gastric emptying, decreased peristalsis; and reduced enteral absorption of water, minerals, and electrolytes.* Because of gut dysfunction secondary to hypoalbuminemia, these PWAs rarely tolerate an oral diet or an intact protein, nasointestinal enteral diet initially. Instead, they must first be treated with either a free amino acid, elemental, nasointestinal, enteral, PPN, or central TPN diet.

Initially, most nutritionists attempt to treat these patients with Vivonex T.E.N., Reabilan HN, or Impact nasointestinal enteral diets. To improve the patient's tolerance of the diets and to reduce diarrhea, they administer plasma expanders, such as albumin 25% or Hespan to increase the serum COP and BWOP, in addition to antidiarrheal agents such as Sandostatin.

As a rule, a serum albumin ≥2.5 g/dL results in a serum COP and BWOP sufficient to maintain normal gut function. Therefore, if the serum albumin is <2.5 g/dL, the albumin deficit is calculated by use of the Andrassy Formula[11, 120]

$$AD = (DSA - ASA) \times 0.3 \times 10 \times wt \ kg^\dagger \qquad 4-2$$

Where AD = albumin deficit (g), DSA = desired serum albumin (2.5 g%), and ASA = Actual serum albumin (g%).
and replaced intravenously by administering 25% albumin, 25 g every 4 to 6 hours. The albumin therapy is continued until the serum albumin is ≥2.5 g/dL.

Because of the cost and the current nationwide shortage of albumin, several nutritionists are now administering Hespan, a synthetic plasma expander (manufactured by Du Pont Pharmaceuti-

---

*References 21, 43–45, 94, 120, 152, 215, 226, 227, 259, 333, 344.

†Hardin T, et al: *Surg Gynecol Obstet* 1989; 163:359. Used by permission.

cals, Wilmington, Del),[244] instead of albumin. Hespan has the same effect as albumin upon serum COP and BWOP. However, in contrast to albumin, Hespan is (1) less expensive, (2) readily available, and (3) associated with fewer side effects. In addition, Hespan, unlike albumin, has no inhibitory effect upon hepatic protein synthesis. The therapeutic dosage of Hespan is variable. The author treats the average 70-kg adult with Hespan 250 cc intravenously over 4 to 6 hours on day 1 of nutritional therapy. If necessary and not contraindicated cardiovascularly, the dosage is repeated on day 2 of therapy.

In addition to the plasma expanders, nutritionists administer antidiarrheal agents to enhance the patient's enteral diet tolerance. In the past, several antidiarrheal agents such as Lomotil, Imodium, and deodorized tincture of opium (DTO) had been used with variable success. Recently, however, the author has successfully used Sandostatin to treat the diarrhea of several PWAs. Currently, the Federal Drug Administration (FDA) has not approved the use of Sandostatin for the treatment of AIDS diarrhea, although it appears to be a very effective antidiarrheal agent.[55] Currently, several clinical trials are under way to evaluate the role of Sandostatin in the treatment of AIDS diarrhea. Hopefully, in the near future, it will be approved by the FDA for the treatment of AIDS diarrhea.

PWAs with a "colitic" enteropathy are initially treated with albumin or Hespan, antidiarrheal agents (e.g., Sandostatin), and Vivonex T.E.N., Reabilan HN, or Impact, full-strength, nasointestinal enteral diets. Patients who fail to tolerate these diets may alternatively be treated with Compleat Modified Formula nasointestinal enteral diet. Patients who tolerate this therapy are later treated according to the "nonspecific" enteropathy nutritional therapy algorithm.

Patients who fail to tolerate enteral diet therapy often require a short course of parenteral diet therapy to correct their nutritional deficiencies, rest the bowel, and facilitate their eventual tolerance of an oral or nasointestinal enteral diet. Patients who require parenteral diet therapy are usually treated with a short course (7 to 10 days) of combined antidiarrheal therapy (e.g., Sandostatin) and PPN therapy. Oral food intake is restricted for several days in an attempt to "rest" the bowel. Frequently, the combination of bowel "rest" plus antidiarrheal and PPN therapy is successful. Patients who experience a significant improvement in the volume and frequency of their diarrhea are later treated according to the "nonspecific" nutritional therapy algorithm.

Patients who do not experience a rapid improvement in the volume and frequency of their diarrhea but who are beginning to display some response after 7 to 10 days of PPN therapy are treated with a short course (>10 days, <3 months) of TPN and continued Sandostatin antidiarrheal therapy. Prior to initiating the TPN therapy, however, the patient should satisfy the criteria previously discussed. By administering a short course (<3 months) of combined TPN and antidiarrheal therapy, the nutritionist can treat the PWA's nutritional deficiencies while the gut dysfunction resolves. Hopefully, after 3 months of TPN therapy, the patient can be treated according to the "nonspecific" enteropathy nutritional therapy algorithm. If not, prolonged (>3 months) TPN therapy is not recommended. The use of prolonged TPN therapy for either intractable diarrhea or oral/enteral diet intolerance is ethically and economically very controversial.* Table 4–9 summarizes the nutritional therapy regimen for PWAs with a "colitic enteropathy."

Cholerrheic Enteropathy Diet

Malnourished PWAs who have watery, large-volume diarrhea and intestinal secretion (i.e., "cholerrheic" enteropathy) are treated according to the same nutritional therapy algorithm as PWAs with a "colitic" enteropathy (see Table 4–9). These patients usually suffer from a chronic cryptosporidiosis, *Mycobacterium avium-intracellulare,* or cytomegalovirus infections that damage the brush border of the intestinal villi. This causes severe physiologic (macronutrient and micronutrient, fluid, and electrolyte malabsorption) and mechanical (intractable diarrhea) gut dysfunction. Fortunately, these infections are periodically active and quiescent. Patients with an active infection have voluminous diarrhea, become severely dehydrated, and develop significant nutritional deficiencies. Therefore, in order to survive, they require antidiarrheal therapy, hydration, and short-term (<3 months) parenteral diet therapy. The treatment algorithm for this group of patients is essentially the same as that for patients with a "colitic" enteropathy with the exclusion of initially attempting a nasointestinal enteral diet. Table 4–9 summarizes the nutritional therapy regimen for PWAs with "cholerrheic" enteropathy.

*References 34, 48, 53, 91, 159, 181, 200, 250, 271, 282, 302, 303, 328.

REFERENCES

1. Abumrad NN, et al: Amino acid and intolerance during prolonged total parenteral nutrition reversed by molybdate therapy. *Am J Clin Nutr* 1981; 34:2551–2559.
2. Alexander JW, et al: Nutritional immuno-modulators in burn patients. *Crit Care Med* 1990; 18:S149–S153.
3. Alexander JW, et al: The importance of lipid type in the diet after burn injury. *Ann Surg* 1986; 204:1–8.
4. Altimari AF, et al: Use of somatostatin analogue (SMS 210-995) in the glucagonoma syndrome. *Surgery* 1986; 100:989–996.
5. Alverdy J, Chi HS, Sheldon GF: The effect of parenteral nutrition on gastrointestinal immunity. The importance of enteral stimulation. *Ann Surg* 1985; 202:681–684.
6. Ament ME, Ochs HD, Davis SD: Structure and function of the gastrointestinal tract in primary immunodeficiency syndrome: A study of 39 patients. *Medicine* 1973; 52:227–248.
7. American Society for Parenteral and Enteral Nutrition, Board of Directors: Guidelines for use of total parenteral nutrition in the hospitalized adult patient. *JPEN* 1986; 10:441–445.
8. American Society for Parenteral and Enteral Nutrition: Care and management of AIDS patients. A.S.P.E.N. 12th Clinical Congress, Las Vegas, Nevada, January 17, 1988.
9. Anderson BJ: Tube feeding: Is diarrhea inevitable? *Am J Nurs* 1986; 704–706.
10. Anderson JV, Bloom SR: Neuroendocrine tumors of the gut: Long-term therapy with the somatostatin analogue SMS 201-995. *Scand J Gastroenterol* 1986; 21(suppl 119):115–128.
11. Andrassy RJ: Enteral elemental nutrition in pediatric surgery. *Contemp Surg* 1986; 28(suppl 4A).
12. Apelgren KN, Wilmore DW: Nutritional care of the critically ill. *Surg Clin North Am* 1983; 63:497–507.
13. Archer DL, Glinsmann WH: Hypothesis: Intestinal infection and malnutrition initiate acquired immune deficiency syndrome (AIDS). *Nutr Res* 5:9–19.
14. Asjo B, Wahren J: Risk of nosocomial AIDS virus infection during intravenous nutrition therapy in AIDS patients: Virus characteristics and precautions. *Nutr Int* 1986; 2:268–270.

15. Awashi YC, Beutler E, Srivastava SK: Purification and properties of human erythrocyte glutathione peroxidase. *J Biol Chem* 1975; 250:5144–5149.

16. Bach MC, et al: Odynophagia from aphthous ulcers of the pharynx and esophagus in the acquired immunodeficiency syndrome (AIDS). *Ann Intern Med* 1988; 109:338–339.

17. Bainton DF, Finch CA: The diagnosis of iron deficiency anemia. *Am J Med* 1964; 37:62.

18. Baker SS, et al: Reversal of biochemical and functional abnormalities in erythrocytes secondary to selenium deficiency. *JPEN* 1983; 7:293–295.

19. Balthazar EJ, et al: Cytomegalovirus, esophagitis and gastritis in AIDS. *AJR* 1985; 144:1201–1204.

20. Barbul A, et al: Arginine stimulates lymphocyte immune response in healthy human beings. *Surgery* 1981; 90:244–251.

21. Barden RP, et al: The influence of serum protein on the motility of the small intestine. *Surgery* 1979; 86:307–315.

22. Barr CE, Torosian JP: Oral manifestations in patients with AIDS or AIDS-related complex (letter). *Lancet* 1986; 2:288.

23. Beach R, Laura P: Nutrition and the acquired immunodeficiency syndrome. *Ann Intern Med* 1983; 99:565–566.

24. Begin ME, Das UN: A deficiency in dietary gamma-linolenic and/or eicosapentaenoic acids may determine individual susceptibility to AIDS. *Med Hypotheses* 1986; 20:1–8.

25. Beisel WR: Metabolic response to infection, in Kinney J, Jeejeebhoy K, Hill G, et al (eds): *Nutrition and Metabolism in Patient Care*. Philadelphia: WB Saunders Co/Harcourt Brace Jovanovich, 1988, p 605.

26. Beisel WR, et al: Single-nutrient effects on immunologic functions. *JAMA* 1981; 245:53–58.

27. Benkov KJ, et al: Atypical presentation of childhood acquired immune deficiency syndrome mimicking Crohn's disease: Nutritional consideration and management. *Am J Gastro Enterol* 1985; 80:260–266.

28. Bennett JA: AIDS beyond the hospital: What we know about AIDS. *Am J Nurs* 1986; 1015–1028.

29. Benson W, et al: Control of watery diarrhea syndrome in a patient with vasoactive intestinal polypeptide-secreting tu-

mor, using SMS 201-995 and dexamethasone. *Scand J Gastroenterol* 1986; 21(suppl 119):107–116.

30. Berk RN, et al: Cryptosporidiosis of the stomach and small intestine in patients with AIDS. *AJR* 1984; 143: 549–554.

31. Beutler B, Cerami A: Cachectin: More than a tumor necrosis factor. *N Engl J Med* 1987; 316:479–485.

32. Beutler B, Milsark IW, Cerami AC: Passive immunization against cachectin/tumor necrosis factor protects mice from lethal effect of endotoxin. *Science* 1985; 229:869–871.

33. Bistrian BR: Interaction of nutrition and infection in the hospital setting. *Am J Clin Nutr* 1977; 30:1228–1232.

34. Bloom DE, Carliner G: The economic impact of AIDS in the United States. *Science* 1988; 239:604–609.

35. Blumberg BS, et al: Iron and iron binding proteins in persistent generalized lymphadenopathy and AIDS. *Lancet* 1984; 1:347–348.

36. Boden G, et al: Treatment of inoperable glucagonoma with the long-acting somatostatin analogue SMS 201-995. *N Engl J Med* 1986; 314:1686–1689.

37. Bothwell TH, Finch CA: *Iron Metabolism*. Boston: Little, Brown & Co, 1962.

38. Bouchard PH: Diabetes mellitus following pentamidine induced hypoglycemia in humans. *Diabetes* 1982; 31: 40–45.

39. Bowen DL, Lane HC, Fauci AS: Cellular immunity, in Ma P, Armstrong D (eds): *The Acquired Immune Deficiency Syndrome and Infections of Homosexual Men*. New York: Medical Books, Technical Publishing, 1984, pp 135–147.

40. Bower RH, Kern KA, Fischer JE: Use of a branched chain amino acid enriched solution in patients under metabolic stress. *Am J Surg* 1985; 149:266–270.

41. Brabant G, et al: Treatment of carcinoid and VIPoma with a long-acting somatostatin analogue (SMS 201-995). *Scand J Gastro Enterol* 1986; 21(suppl 119):117–180.

42. Brinson RR: Hypoalbuminemia, diarrhea and the acquired immunodeficiency syndrome. *Ann Intern Med* 1985; 102:413.

43. Brinson RR, Kolts B: Hypoalbuminemia as an indicator of diarrheal incidence in critically ill patients. *Crit Care Med* May 1987; 15:506–509.

44. Brinson RR, Curtis WD, Singh M: Diarrhea in the inten-

sive care unit. The role of hypoalbuminemia and the response to a peptide-based diet. *J Am Coll Nutr* 1987; 15:506.

45. Brinson RR, et al: Hypoalbuminemia-associated diarrhea in critically ill patients. *J Crit Ill* 1987.

46. Brinson RR, et al: Intestinal absorption of peptide enteral formulas in hypoproteinemic (volume expanded) rats: A paired analysis. *Crit Care Med* 1989; 17:657–660.

47. Bro S, et al: Serum zinc in homosexual men with antibodies against human immunodeficiency virus. *Clin Chem* 1988; 34:1929–1930.

48. Brolin RE, et al: Use of nutrition support in patients with AIDS. Unpublished manuscript from Department of Surgery, UMDNJ-Robert Wood Johnson Medical School and Nutrition Support Team at Robert Wood Johnson University Hospital, New Brunswick, NJ, 1988.

49. Budd CB: Nutritional care of patients with *Pneumocystis carinii* pneumonia. *Nutr Suppl Serv* 1982; 2:12–13.

50. Burch RE, Hahn HKJ: Trace elements in human nutrition. *Med Clin North Am* 1979; 63:1057–1058.

51. Burroughs Wellcome Co, Product Development Information: Important information about retrovir: Development, efficacy and safety, 1987.

52. Buzby GP, et al: Prognostic nutritional index in gastrointestinal surgery. *Am J Surg* 1980; 139:160–167.

53. California Medical Association Council: Withholding or withdrawing life-sustaining treatment: Ethical guidelines for decision making in long-term care facilities. January 17, 1986.

54. Cathcart RF: Vitamin C in the treatment of acquired immunodeficiency syndrome (AIDS). *Med Hypotheses* 1984; 18:61–77.

55. Cello JP, et al: Controlled clinical trial of octreotide for refractory AIDS-associated diarrhea. Abstract 163 presented at the American Digestive Week Meeting, San Antonio, Tex, May 1990.

56. Centers for Disease Control: Revision of the CDC surveillance case, definition for acquired immunodeficiency syndrome. *MMWR* 1987; 35(suppl 1S):3S–15S.

57. Centers for Disease Control: Revision of the CDC surveillance case, definition for acquired immunodeficiency syndrome. MMWR, 1987; 35(suppl 1S):3S–15S. Update: Ac-

quired immunodeficiency syndrome; United States. *MMWR* 1984; 32:688–691.

58. Cerra FB, et al: Cardiac beta-adrenergic responsiveness is well preserved in moderate protein calorie malnutrition from semistarvation. *JPEN* 1988; 12:635–675.

59. Cerra FB, et al: Septic autocannibalism. A failure of exogenous nutritional support. *Ann Surg* 1980; 192:570–580.

60. Ch'ng JL, et al: Remission of symptoms during long-term treatment of metastatic pancreatic endocrine tumors with long-acting somatostatin analogue. *Br J Med* [Clin Res] 1985; 2:981–982.

61. Chandra RK: Excessive intake of zinc impairs immune response. *JAMA* 1984; 252:1443–1447.

62. Chandra RK: Immune response to parasites. B. Mechanisms. *Rev Infect Dis* 1982; 4:756–762.

63. Chandra RK: Immunocompetence in undernutrition. *J Pediatr* 1972; 81:1194–1200.

64. Chandra RK: Immunocompetence is a functional index of nutritional status. *Br Med Bull* 1981; 37:89–94.

65. Chandra RK: *Immunology of Nutritional Disorders*. London, Arnold, 1980.

66. Chandra RK: Mucosal immune responses to malnutrition. *Ann NY Acad Sci* 1983; 409:345–352.

67. Chandra RK: Nutrition and immunity-basic considerations, part 1. *Contemp Nutr* 1986; 11:11.

68. Chandra RK: The nutrition-immunity nexus: The enumeration and functional assessment of lymphocyte subsets in nutritional deficiency. *Nutr Res* 1983; 3:605–616.

69. Chandra RK: Nutrition, immunity and infection: Present knowledge and future directions. *Lancet* 1983; 1:688–691.

70. Chandra RK: Parasite infection, nutrition and immune response. *Fed Proc* 1984; 43:251–255.

71. Chandra RK: Serum complement and immunoconglutinin in malnutrition. *Arch Dis Child* 1975; 50:225–229.

72. Chandra RK, Dayton DH: Trace element regulation of immunity and infection. *Nutr Res* 1982; 2:721–733.

73. Chandra RK, Newberne PM: *Nutrition, Immunity and Infection: Mechanisms of Interaction*. New York: Plenum Publishing Corp, 1977.

74. Chandra RK, Puri S: Trace element modulation of immune responses, in Chandra RK (ed): *Trace Elements*. New York: Raven, 1985.

75. Chandra RK, et al: Iron status, immunocompetence and susceptibility to infection, in *Iron Metabolism*. Ciba Foundation Symposium No. 51. Amsterdam, Elsevier, 1977, pp 249–268.

76. Chandra RK, et al: Nutrition and immunocompetence of the elderly. Effect of short-term nutritional supplementation on cell-mediated immunity and lymphocyte subsets. *Nutr Res* 1982; 2:223–232.

77. Chlebowski RT: Significance of altered nutritional status in acquired immunodeficiency syndrome (AIDS). *Nutr Cancer* 1985; 7:86–89.

78. Clements D, et al: Regression of metastatic VIPoma with somatostatin analogue SMS 201-295. *Lancet* 1985; 1:874–875.

79. Clinical Nutrition Cases: Severe malnutrition in a young man with AIDS. *Nutr Rev* 1988; 46:126–132.

80. Colman N, Grossman F: Nutritional factors in epidemic Kaposi's sarcoma. *Semin Oncol* 1987; 14:54–62.

81. Cone LA, et al: An update on the acquired immunodeficiency syndrome (AIDS) associated disorders of the alimentary tract. *Dis Colon Rectum* 1986; 29:60–63.

82. Cook DJ, et al: Somatostatin treatment for cryptosporidial diarrhea in a patient with acquired immunodeficiency syndrome (AIDS). *Ann Intern Med* 1988; 108:708–709.

83. Cooper JC, et al: Effects of a long-acting somatostatin analogue in patients with severe ileostomy diarrhea. *Br J Surg* 1986; 73:128–131.

84. Cotzias GC: Trace subst. environ. Health-Proc Mo. 1st Annual Conference, 1967, p 5.

85. Cryer A, Bartley W: Studies on the adaptation of rates to a diet high in glycerol. *Int J Biochem* 1973; 4:293–308.

86. Cryptosporidiosis: Assessment of chemotherapy of males with acquired immunodeficiency syndrome (AIDS). *MMWR* 1982; 31:589–592.

87. Cunningham-Rundles S: Effects of nutritional status on immunologic function. *Am J Clin Nutr* 1982; 35:1202–1210.

88. Cunningham-Rundles S, et al: Zinc deficiency depressed

thymic hormones and T-lymphocyte dysfunction in patients with hypogammaglobulinemia. *Clin Immunol Immunopathol* 1983; 21:387–396.

89. Curran JW, et al: Epidemiology of HIV infection and AIDS in the United States. *Science* 1988; 239:610–616.

90. Current WL, et al: Human cryptosporidiosis in immunocompetent and immunodeficient persons: Studies of an outbreak and experimental transmission. *N Engl J Med* 1983; 308:1252–1257.

91. Current Opinions of the Council on Ethical and Judicial Affairs of the American Medical Association—1986. Withholding or withdrawing life-prolonging medical treatment. Chicago, American Medical Association, 1986.

92. Daly JM, et al: Immune and metabolic effects of arginine in the surgical patient. *Ann Surg* 1988; 208:512–522.

93. Dharmsathaphorn K, et al: Somatostatin decreases diarrhea in patients with short bowel syndrome. *J Clin Gastroenterol* 1982; 4:521–524.

94. Diamond JM: Osmotic water flow in leaky epithelia. *J Membr Biol* 1979; 51:195–216.

95. Dilley JW, et al: Findings in psychiatric consultations with patients with acquired immunodeficiency syndrome. *Am J Psychiatry* 1985; 142:82–86.

96. Domaldo TL, et al: Nutritional management of patients with AIDS and cryptosporidium infection. *Nutr Support Serv* 1986; 6:30–31.

97. Dueno Mi, et al: Effect of somatostatin analogue on water and electrolyte transport and transit time in human small bowel. *Dig Dis Sci* 1987; 32:1092–1096.

98. Duran M, et al: Combined deficiency of xanthine oxidase and sulphite oxidase: A defect of molybdenum metabolism or transport? *J Inherited Metab Dis* 1978; 1:175–178.

99. Dworkin BM, et al: Gastrointestinal manifestations of the acquired immunodeficiency syndrome: A review of 22 cases. *Am J Gastroenterol* 1985; 80:774–778.

100. Dworkin BM, et al: Selenium deficiency in the acquired immunodeficiency syndrome. *JPEN* 1986; 10:405–407.

101. Edwards OM, et al: Urinary creatinine excretions as an index of the completeness of 24-hour urine collections. *Lancet* 1969; 2:1165.

102. El-Dadr W, Simberkoff MS: Survival and prognostic factors in severe *Pneumocystis carinii* pneumonia requiring

mechanical ventilation. *Am Rev Respir Dis* 1988; 137:1264–1267.

103. Elia M, et al: Clinical usefulness of urinary 3-methylhistidine excretion in indicating muscle protein breakdown. *Br Med J* 1981; 282:3511–3540.

104. Ellison EC, et al: Modulation of functional gastrointestinal endocrine tumors by endogenous and exogenous somatostatin. *Am J Surg* 1986; 151:668–675.

105. Fabris N, et al: AIDS, zinc deficiency and thymic hormone failure. *JAMA* 1988; 259:839–840.

106. Fairclough PD, et al: New evidence for intact di- and tripeptide absorption. *Gut* 1975; 16:843a.

107. Fairclough PD, et al: A comparison of the absorption of two protein hydrolysates and their effects on water and electrolyte movements in the human jejunum. *Gut* 1980; 21:829.

108. Fairfull-Smith RJ, et al: Use of glycerol in peripheral parenteral nutrition. *Surgery* 1982; 91:728–732.

109. Falutz J, Tsoukas C, Gold C: Zinc in human immunodeficiency virus infection. Reply (letter). *JAMA* 1988; 260:1882.

110. Falutz J, et al: Zinc deficiency and human immunodeficiency virus infection. *Clin Invest Med* 1987; 10:B49.

111. Fanslow KC, et al: Effect of nucleotide restriction and supplementation on resistance to experimental nurine candidiasis. *JPEN* 1988; 12:49–52.

112. Fedorak RN, Field M: Antidiarrheal therapy. Prospects for new agents. *Dig Dis Sci* 1987; 32:192–205.

113. Fell GS, Halls D, Shenkin A: in Shapcott D, Hubert J (eds): *Chromium in Nutrition and Metabolism*. New York: Elsevier, North-Holland, 1979, 105–111.

114. Felsenstein D, et al: Treatment of cytomegalovirus retinitis with 9-[2-hydroxyl-1-(hydroxymethyl) ethoxymethyl] guanine. *Ann Intern Med* 1985; 103:377–380.

115. Fernandes G, et al: Impairment of cell-mediated immunity functions by dietary zinc deficiency in mice. *Proc Natl Acad Sci USA* 1979; 76:457–461.

116. Fiasse R, et al: Short-term effects of the long-acting somatostatin analogue SMS 201-995 in five cases of APUDoma (four with metastases) and in one case of systemic macrocytosis. *Scand J Gastroenterol* 1986; 21(suppl 119):212–216.

117. Fleming CR: Selenium deficiency and fatal cardiomyopathy in a patient on home parenteral nutrition. *Gastroenterology* 1982; 83:689–693.

118. Fleming CR, Nelson J: Nutritional options, in Kinney J, Jeejeebhoy K, Hill G, et al (eds): *Nutrition and Metabolism in Patient Care*. Philadelphia: WB Saunders Co/Harcourt Brace Jovanovich, 1988, p 752.

119. Food and Nutrition Board: *Recommended Daily Dietary Allowances,* ed 9., Washington, DC: National Academy of Sciences, National Research Council, 1980.

120. Ford EG, Andrassy RJ: Serum albumin (oncotic pressure) correlates with enteral feeding tolerance in the pediatric surgical patient. *J Pediatr Surg* 1987; 22:597–599.

121. Frank D, Raicht RF: Intestinal perforation associated with cytomegalovirus infection in patients with acquired immunodeficiency syndrome. *Am J Gastroenterol* 1984; 79:201–205.

122. Frankel AD, Bredt DS, Pabo CO: Tat-III protein from HIV forms and metal-linked dimer. *J Cell Biochem* 1988; (suppl 0 [12 part D]):322.

123. Freeman JB, et al: Safety and efficacy of a new peripheral intravenously administered amino acid solution containing glycerol and electrolytes. *Surg Gynecol Obstet* 1983; 156:625–631.

124. Freund H, Atamian S, Fischer JE: Chromium deficiency during total parenteral nutrition. *JAMA* 1979; 241:496–497.

125. Fuessl HS, et al: Effects of a long-acting somatostatin analogue (SMS 201-995) on postprandial gastric emptying of Tc-tin colloid and mouth-to-caecum transit time in man. *Digestion* 1987; 36:101–107.

126. Fuessl HS, et al: Symptomatic treatment of uncontrollable diarrhea in AIDS with the Somatostatin Analog SMS 201-995. *Klin Wochenschr* 1988; 66(suppl 13):240–241.

127. Fuessl HS, et al: Treatment of secretory diarrhea in AIDS with the Somatostatin Analog SMS 201-295. *Klin Wochenschr* 1989; 67:452–455.

128. Gaginella TS, O'Dorisio TM: Octreotide: Entering the new era of peptidomimetic therapy. *Drug Intell Clin Pharm* 1988; 22:154–155.

129. Garcia ME, Collins CL, Mansell PWA: The acquired immune deficiency syndrome: Nutational complication and

assessment of body weight status. *Nutr Clin Pract* 1987; 2:108–111.

130. Geelhoed GW, et al: Somatostatin analogue: Effects on hypergastrinemia and hypercalcitoninemia. *Surgery* 1986; 100:962–970.

131. Gelb A, Miller S: AIDS and gastroenterology. *Am J Gastro Enterol* 1986; 81:619–621.

132. Gerberding JL, et al: The risk of transmitting the human immunodeficiency virus, cytomegalovirus and hepatitis B virus to health care workers exposed to patients with AIDS and AIDS-related conditions. *J Infect Dis* 1987; 156:27–28.

133. Gertler SL, et al: Gastrointestinal cytomegalovirus infection in a homosexual man with severe acquired immunodeficiency syndrome. *Gastroenterology* 1983; 85:1403–1406.

134. Gillin JS, et al: Disseminated mycobacterium avium-intracellular infection in acquired immunodeficiency syndrome mimicking Whipple's disease. *Gastroenterology* 1983; 85:1187–1191.

135. Gillin JS, et al: Malabsorption and mucosal abnormalities of the small intestine in the acquired immunodeficiency syndrome. *Ann Inter Med* 1985; 102:619–622.

136. Goldman DW, Pickett WC, Goetzl EJ: Human neutrophil chemotactic and degranulating activities of leukotriene B5 derived from eicosapentaenoic acid. *Biochem Biophys Res Commun* 1983; 117:282.

137. Goldsmith GA: Trace element regulation of immunity and infection. *J Am Coll Nutr* 1985; 51:727–733.

138. Good RA: Nutrition and immunity. *J Clin Immunol* 1981; 1:3–9.

139. Good RA, et al: Influence of nutrition on antibody production and cellular immune responses in man, rats, mice and guinea pigs. in Suskind RM (ed): *Malnutrition and the Immune Response*. New York: Raven, 1977, pp 169–183.

140. Good RA, et al: Nutritional deficiency, immunologic function and disease. *Am J Pathol* 1979; 84:599–614.

141. Goodhart R, Shils M: *Modern Nutrition in Health and Disease,* ed 5. Philadelphia: Lea & Febiger, 1988, p 821.

142. Goodman AG, Gilman L: *The Pharmacological Basis of Therapeutics,* ed 7. New York: Macmillan Publishing Co, 1985.

143. Gottleib MS, et al: *Pneumocystis carinii* pneumonia and mucosal candidiasis in previously healthy homosexual men;

evidence of a new acquired cellular immunodeficiency. *N Engl J Med* 1981; 305:1425–1431.

144. Granger DN, Brinson RR: Intestinal absorption of elemental and standard enteral formulas in hypoproteinemic (volume expanded) rats. *JPEN* 1988; 12:278.

145. Grant JP, et al: Current techniques of nutritional assessment. *Surg Clin North Am* 1981; 61:437–463.

146. Gray RH: Similarities between AIDS and PCM (letter). *Am J Public Health* 1983; 73:1332.

147. Guidelines for essential trace element preparations for parenteral use. Expert Panel for Nutrition Advisory Group, AMA Department of Foods and Nutrition. *JAMA* 1979; 241:2051.

148. Guinan ME, Hardy A: Epidemiology of AIDS in women in the United States. *JAMA* 1987; 257:2039–2042.

149. Gupta S, et al: Serum ferritin in acquired immunodeficiency syndrome. *J Clin Lab* 1986; 20:11–13.

150. Hagen JH: The effect of insulin on concentration of plasma glycerol. *J Lipid Res* 1963; 4:46–51.

151. Hankins DA, et al: Whole blood trace element concentrations during total parenteral nutrition. *Surgery* 1976; 79:674–677.

152. Hardin TC, Page CP, Schweisinger WH: Rapid replacement of serum albumin in patients receiving total parenteral nutrition. *Surg Gynecol Obstet* 1986; 163:359–362.

153. Harriman GR, et al: Vitamin B12 malabsorption in patients with acquired immunodeficiency syndrome. *Clin Res* 1987; 35:409A.

154. Hegarty JE, et al: Effects of concentration on in vivo absorption of a peptide containing protein hydrolysate. *Gut* 1982; 23:304.

155. Higgins ES, Reichert DA, Westerfield WW: Molybdate deficiency and tungsten inhibition studies. *J Nutr* 1956; 59:539–559.

156. Hitzig WH: The Swiss type of agammaglobulinemia, in Good RA, Bergsma D (eds): *Immunologic Deficiencies in Man,* (volume 4 of Birth Defects: Original Article Series), New York: National Foundation, 1968, pp 82–87.

157. Hoff R, et al: Seroprevalence of human immunodeficiency virus among childbearing women. *N Engl J Med* 1988; 318:525–530.

158. Hopewell PC, Luce JM: Pulmonary involvement in the acquired immunodeficiency syndrome. *Chest* 1985; 87:104–112.

159. Hughes A, Martin J, Franks P: AIDS home care and hospice manual: AIDS home care and hospice program. San Francisco, Visiting Nurses Association of San Francisco, 1987.

160. Hutchins KC: Thiamine deficiency, Wernicke's encephalopathy and AIDS. *Lancet* 1987; 23:2100.

161. Islikar H, Schurch B: *The Impact of Malnutrition on Immune Defense in Parasitic Infestation.* Islikar H Schurch B, eds. Bern: Hans Stuber, 1981.

162. Jacobsen S, Wester PO: Balance studies of twenty trace elements during total parenteral nutrition in man. *Br J Med* 37:107–126.

163. Jain VK, Chandra RK: Does nutritional deficiency predispose to acquired immunodeficiency syndrome? *Nutr Reas* 1984; 4:537–543.

164. Jaros W, et al: Successful treatment of idiopathic secretory diarrhea of infancy with the somatostatin analogue SMS 201-995. *Gastroenterology* 1988; 94:189–193.

165. Jeejeebhoy KN, et al: Chromium deficiency, glucose intolerance and neuropathy reversed by chromium supplementation in a patient receiving long-term total parenteral nutrition. *Am J Clin Nutr* 1977; 30:531.

166. Johnson JL, Rajagopalan KV, Cohen HJ: Molecular basis of the biologic function of molybdenum: Effect of tungsten on xanthine oxidase and sulfite oxidase in the rat. *J Biol Chem* 1974; 249:859–866.

167. Johnson IL, et al: Inborn errors of molybdenum metabolism: Combined deficiencies of sulfite oxidase and xanthine dehydrogenase in a patient lacking the molybdenum cofactor. *Proc Natl Acad Sci USA* 1980; 77:3715–3719.

168. Jordon B, et al: Neurological syndromes complicating AIDS. *Front Radiat Ther Oncol* 1985; 19:82–87.

169. Kaihara S, Wagner HN Jr: Measurement of intestinal fat absorption with carbon-14 labeled tracers. *J Lab Clin Med,* 1968; 71:400–411.

170. Katz MD, Erstad B: Octreotide, a new somatostatin analogue. *Clin Pharm* 1989; 8:225–273.

171. Katz MD, et al: Treatment of severe cryptosporidium-

related diarrhea with octreotide in a patient with AIDS. *Drug Intell Clin Pharm* 1988; 22:134–136.

172. Keohane PP, et al: The peptide nitrogen source of elemental diets—effects of peptide chain length on absorptive characteristics. A.S.P.E.N., 7th Clinical Conference (abstract). *JPEN* 1983; 6:23–28.

173. Keusch CT, et al: Humoral and cellular aspects of intracellular bacteria killing in Guatemalan children with protein-calorie malnutrition, in RM Suskind RM (ed): *Malnutrition and the Immune Response.* New York; Raven, 1977, pp 245–251.

174. Kotler DP: Diarrhea in AIDS—diagnosis and management. *Res Staff Phys* 1987; 33:30–41.

175. Khalidi N: Trace elements: An update. *Nutr Suppl Serv* 1988; 8:22–24.

176. Kien EL, Ganthor HZ: Manifestations of chronic selenium deficiency in a child receiving total parenteral nutrition. *Am J Clin Nutr* 1984; 37:319–321.

177. Klein RS, et al: Oral candidiasis in high risk patients at the initial manifestations of the acquired immunodeficiency syndrome. *N Engl J Med* 1984; 311:354–358.

178. Knapp AB, et al: Widespread cytomegalovirus gastroenterocolitis in a patient with acquired immunodeficiency syndrome. *Gastroenterology* 1983; 85:1399–1402.

179. Koch KL, et al: Cryptosporidiosis in a patient with hemophilia, common variable hypogammaglobulinemia and the acquired immunodeficiency syndrome. *Ann Intern Med* 1983; 99:337–340.

180. Koelz A, et al: Escape of response to a long-acting somatostatin analogue (SMS 201-995) in patients with VIPoma. *Gastroenterology* 1987; 92:527–531.

181. Kotler D: Nutrition therapy held possibly lifesaving. *Med Tribune,* November 9, 1989.

182. Kotler DP: Why study nutrition in AIDS? *Nutr Clin Pract* 1987; 1:94–95.

183. Kotler DP, Wang J, Pierson RN: Body composition studies in patients with acquired immunodeficiency syndrome. *Am J Clin Nutr* 1985; 42:1255–1265.

184. Kotler DP, et al: Enteropathy associated with the acquired immunodeficiency syndrome. *Ann Intern Med* 1984; 101:421–428.

185. Kovacevic Z, McGivan JD: Mitochondrial metabolism of

glutamine and glutamate and its physiological significance. *Physiol Rev* 1983; 63:547–605.

186. Krejs GJ, Browne R, Raskin P: Effect of intravenous somatostatin on jejunal absorption of glucose, amino acids, water and electrolytes. *Gastroenterology* 1980; 78:26–31.

187. Kulkarni AD, et al: Influence of dietary nucleotide restriction on bacterial sepsis and phagocytic cell function in mice. *Arch Surg* 1986; 121:169–172.

188. Kvols LK, et al: The treatment of the malignant carcinoid syndrome—evaluation of a long-acting somatostatin analogue. *N Engl J Med* 1986; 315:663–666.

189. Kvols LK, et al: The treatment of metastatic islet cell carcinoma with a somatostatin analogue (SMS 201-995). *Ann Intern Med* 1987; 107:162–168.

190. Lahdevirta J, et al: Elevated levels of circulatory cachectin/tumor necrosis factor in patients with acquired immunodeficiency syndrome. *Am J Med* 1988; 85:289–291.

191. Lane HC, et al: Abnormalities of B-cell activation and immunoregulation in patients with the acquired immunodeficiency syndrome. *N Engl J Med* 1983; 309:453–458.

192. Lasser KM, Lwein KJ, Rynning FW: Cryptosporidial enteritis in a patient with congenital hypogammaglobulinemia. *Hum Pathol* 1979; 10:234–240.

193. Lee TH, et al: Effect of dietary enrichment with eicosapentaenoic acids in vitro neutrophil and monocyte leukotriene generation and neutrophil function. *N Engl J Med* 1985; 312:1217.

194. Leoung GS, et al: Dapsone-trimethoprim for *Pneumocystis carinii* pneumonia in the acquired immunodeficiency syndrome. *Ann Intern Med* 1986; 105:45–48.

195. Levander OA: Selenium: Biochemical actions, interactions and some human health implications, in *Clinical, Biochemical and Nutritional Aspects of Trace Elements*. New York: Alan R. Liss, 1982, pp 345–368.

196. Levander OA, et al: Selenium balance in young men during selenium depletion and repletion. *Am J Clin Nutr* 1981; 34:2662–2669.

197. Lieberman MD, et al: Effects of nutrient substrates on immune function. *Nutrition* 1990; 6:88–91.

198. Lokesh BR, Hsieh HL, Kinsella JE: Peritoneal macrophages from mice fed dietary (w-3) polyunsaturated fatty acids secrete low levels of prostaglandins. *J Nutr* 1986; 116:2547.

199. Lowery SF, et al: Whole body protein breakdown and 3-methylhistidine excretion during brief fasting, starvation and intravenous repletion in man. *Ann Surg* 1985; 202:21–27.

200. Luce JM, Wachter RM, Hopewell PC: Intensive care of patients with the acquired immunodeficiency syndrome: Time for a reassessment? (editorial). *Am Rev Respir Dis* 1988; 137:1261–1263.

201. Magrum LJ, Johnstone PV: Effect of culture in vitro with eicosatetraenoic and eicosapentaenoic acids in fatty acid composition, prostaglandin synthesis and chemiluminescence of rat peritoneal macrophages. *Biochem Biophys Acta* 836, 1984; 836:354.

202. Malebranche R, et al: Acquired immunodeficiency syndrome with severe gastrointestinal manifestations in Haiti. *Lancet* 1983; 2:873–878.

203. March HM, et al: Carcinoid crisis during anesthesia: Successful treatment with a somatostatin analogue. *Anesthesiology* Vol. 66, 1987, pp. 89–91.

204. Mark DA, Baliga BS, Suskind RM: Vitamin A deficiency and T-cell immunocompetence (abstract). *Fed Proc* 1989; 39:341.

205. Mascioli EA, et al: Endotoxin challenge after menhaden oil diet: Effects on survival of guinea pigs. *Am J Clin Nutr* 1989; 49:277–282.

206. Mascioli EA, et al: Enhanced survival to endoxin in guinea pigs fed i.v. fish oil. *Lipids* 1988; 23:623–625.

207. Mass L, Grochowski J: in *Medical Answers About AIDS*, Grochowski J (ed): New York: GMHC Publications, 1987.

208. Masur H, et al: An outbreak of community-acquired *Pneumocystis carinii* pneumonia: Initial manifestation of cellular immune dysfunction. *N Engl J Med* 1981; 305:1431–1438.

209. Maton PN, et al: Use of somatostatin and somatostatin analogues in a patient with glucagonoma. *J Clin Endocrinol Metab* 1981; 53:543–549.

210. McCaffrey EA: Meeting nutritional needs: Stimulating appetite and maximizing caloric intake. *AIDS Patient Care* 1987; 1:28–31.

211. McCarthy DP, Kluger MJ, Vander AJ: Suppression of food intake during infection: Is interleukin-1 involved? *Am J Clin Nutr* 1985; 42:1179–1182.

212. McClain CJ: Trace metal abnormalities in adults during hyperalimentation. *JPEN* 1981; 5:424–429.

213. McConnell KP, et al: Selenium levels in human blood and tissues in health and disease. *J Nutr* 1975; 106:1026–1031.

214. McLean APH, Meakins JL: Nutritional support in sepsis. *Surg Clin North Am* 1981; 61:681–690.

215. Meguid MM, et al: Effect of enteral diet on albumin and urea-synthesis: Comparison with partially hydrolyzed protein diet. *J Surg Res* 1981; 37:16–24.

216. Meisel JL, et al: Overwhelming watery diarrhea associated with cryptosporidium in an immunosuppressed patient. *Gastroenterology* 1975; 70:1156–1160.

217. Meiselman MS, Cello JP, Margaretten W: Cytomegalovirus colitis. *Gastroenterology* 1985; 88:171–175.

218. Mercure L, et al: Inhibition of the AIDS virus replication by a long-acting Somatostatin analog (abstract 3548). in *Fourth International Conference on AIDS*. Stockholm, June 12–16, 1988, Book II, p 153.

219. Miller RM, et al: Skeletal changes of copper deficiency in infants receiving prolonged total parenteral nutrition. *J Pediatr* 1980; 92:947–949.

220. Mitchell GF: T-cell dependent effect in parasitic infection and disease, in Fougereau M Dausett J (eds): *Immunology 80*. London; Academic, 1980, pp 794–808.

221. Modigliani R, et al: Diarrhea and malabsorption in acquired immunodeficiency syndrome: A study of four cases with special emphasis on opportunistic protozoan infestations. *Gut* 1985; 26:179–187.

222. Molla AM, et al: Rice powder electrolyte solution as oral therapy in diarrhea due to vibro cholerae and *Escherichia coli*. *Lancet* 1982; 1:1317–1319.

223. Moller N, et al: Effects of the somatostatin analogue SMS 201-995 (Sandostatin) on mouth-to-caecum transit time and absorption of fat and carbohydrates in normal man. *Clin Sci* 1988; 75:345–350.

224. Moseson M: Nutrition and AIDS. *Nutr Res* 1986; 6:729–730.

225. Moss G: Malabsorption associated with extreme malnutrition: Importance of replacing plasma albumin. *J Am Coll Nutr* 1982; 1:89–92.

226. Moss G: Plasma albumin and postoperative ileus. *Surg Forum* 1967; 18:333.

227. Moss G, Braunstein FM, Newkirk RE: Postoperative enteral hyperalimentation for cryptosporidial acute cholecystitis associated with AIDS and enteritis. *J Am Coll Nutr* 1987; 6:351–353.

228. Muth OH: White muscle disease, a selenium-responsive myopathy. *J Am Vet Med Assoc* 1963; 142:272–277.

229. National Dairy Council: Nutrition and the immune response. *Dairy Council Dig* 1985; 56:7–12.

230. Navia BA, et al: The AIDS dementia complex: Clinical features. *Ann Neurol* 1986; 19:517–525.

231. Neumann CG, et al: Immunologic responses in malnourished children. *Am J Clin Nutr* 1975; 28:89–104.

232. Nichols SE: Psychiatric aspects of AIDS. *Psychosomatics* 1983; 24:1083–1089.

233. Nime FA, et al: Acute enterocolitis in a human being infected with the protozoan cryptosporidium. *Gastroenterology* 1976; 70:592–598.

234. O'Conner CR, O'Dorisio TM: Amyloidosis, diarrhea and a somatostatin analogue. *Ann Intern Med* 1989; 110:665–666.

235. O'Sullivan P, Line RA, Dalton S: Evaluation of body weight and nutritional status among AIDS patients. *J Am Diet Assoc* 1985; 84:1483–1484.

236. Oberg K, et al: The effects of octreotide on basal and stimulated hormone levels in patients with carcinoid syndrome. *J Clin Endocrinol Metab* 1989; 68:796–800.

237. Oliff A, et al: Tumors secreting human TNF/cachectin induce cachexia in mice. *Cell* 1987; 50:555–563.

238. Ortiz R, Betancourt M: Cell proliferation in bone marrow cells of severely malnourished animals. *J Nutr* 1984, 114:472–476.

239. Osei K, et al: Malignant insulinoma: Effects of a somatostatin analogue (compound SMS 201-995) on serum glucose, growth and gastroenteropancreatic hormones. *Ann Intern Med* 1985; 103:223–225.

240. Patton JS, et al: Interferons and tumor necrosis factors have similar catabolic effects on 3T3 L1 cells. *Proc Natl Acad Sci USA* 1986; 83:8313–8317.

241. Pemberton LB, et al: Sepsis from triple vs. single-lumen catheters during total parenteral nutrition in surgical or critically ill patients. *Arch Surg* 1986; 121:591–594.

242. Perry S, Jacobsen P: Neuropsychiatric manifestations of AIDS—spectrum disorders. *Hosp Community Psychiatr* 1986; 37:135–142.

243. Phelan JA, et al: Oral findings in patients with acquired immunodeficiency syndrome. *Oral Surg Oral Med Oral Pathol* 1988; 64:50–56.

244. *Physicians' Desk Reference,* ed 44. Barnhart ER, ed. Oradell, NJ: Medical Economics Company, 1990.

245. Pine RW: The triple-lumen central venous catheter. *Nutrition in Clinical Practice.* Silver Spring, Md: A.S.P.E.N., 1986.

246. Pleban PA, Munyani A, Beachum J: Determination of selenium concentration and glutathione peroxidase activity in plasma and erythrocytes. *Clin Chem* 1982; 28:311–316.

247. Portnoy D, Whiteside M, Buckley E: Treatment of intestinal cryptosporidiosis with spiramycin. *Ann Intern Med* 1984; 101:202–204.

248. Prasad A: Nutritional zinc today. *Nutr Today* 1981; 16:4–11.

249. Prasad AS: *Trace Elements and Iron in Human Metabolism.* New York: Plenum Publishing Corp, 1978.

250. President's Commission for the Study of Ethical Problems in Medicine and Biomedical and Behavioral Research. Deciding to forego "life-sustaining" treatment: A report on the ethical, medical and legal issues in treatment decisions. Washington, DC, Government Printing Office, 1983.

251. Reichert DA, Westerfield WW: Isolation and identification of xanthine oxidase factor as molybdenum. *J Biol Chem* 1953; 203:915–923.

252. Rene E, et al: Somatostatin and cryptosporidial diarrhea during AIDS (abstract 252). *Can J Physiol Pharmacol* 1986; 70(suppl).

253. Richie E, Copeland EM: Relationship between nutrition and immunity: An overview. *Cancer Bull* 1978; 30:78–84.

254. Richmond J, Girdwood R: Observations on amino acid absorption. *Clin Sci* 1962; 22:301.

255. Roberts WG, Fedorak RN, Chang EB: In vitro effects of long-acting somatostatin analogue SMS 201-995 on electrolyte transport by the rabbit ileum. *Gastroenterology* 1988; 94:1343–1350.

256. Robinson EN, Fuegel R: SMS 201-995, a Somatostatin

analogue and diarrhea in the acquired immunodeficiency syndrome (AIDS). *Ann Intern Med* 1988; 109:680–681.

257. Rodgers VD, Kagnoff MF: Gastrointestinal manifestations of the acquired immunodeficiency syndrome. *West J Med* 1987; 146:57–67.

258. Rodgers VD, Fassett R, Kagnoff MF: Abnormalities in intestinal mucosa T-cells in homosexual populations including those with lymphadenopathy syndrome and acquired immunodeficiency syndrome. *Gastroenterology* Vol. 1986; 90:552–558.

259. Rombeau JL, Caldwell MD: Enteral and tube feeding, in *Clinical Nutrition,* vol I. Philadelphia: WB Saunders Co, 1984.

260. Rosen FS: The thymus gland and the immune deficiency syndromes, in Sumter M (ed): *Immunological Diseases*. vol 1.Boston: Little, Brown & Co, 1971, pp 497–519.

261. Rosen MJ, Cucco RA, Teirstein AS: Outcome of intensive care in patients with acquired immunodeficiency syndrome. *J Intensive Care Med* 1986; 1:55–60.

262. Ross IN, Asquith P: Primary immune therapy deficiency, in Asquith P (ed): *Immunology of the Gastrointestinal Tract*. Edinburgh: Churchill Livingstone, 1979, pp 152–182.

263. Roth RI, Owen R, Keren DF: AIDS with *Mycobacterium avium-intracellular* lesions resembling those of Whipple's disease (letter). *N Engl J Med* 1983; 309:1324.

264. Rubin RH: Acquired immunodeficiency syndrome, in Rubenstein E, Federmann DD (eds): *Scientific American Medicine*. New York: Scientific American Inc, 1987.

265. Saito H, et al: Metabolic and immune effects of dietary arginine supplementation after burn. *Arch Surg* 1987; 122:784–789.

266. Salonen JT, et al: Risk of cancer in relation to serum concentrations of selenium and vitamins A and E: Matched case-control analysis of prospective data. *Br Med J [Clin Sci]* 1985; 290:417–420.

267. Santos JI, Arrendondo JL, Vitale JJ: Nutrition, infection and immunity. *Pediatr Ann* 1983; 12:182–194.

268. Sato SJ, Mirtallo JM: Nutritional support for the AIDS patient. *US Pharm* 1987; H2–H9.

269. Saxena QB, Saxena RK, Adler WH: Effect of protein calorie malnutrition on the levels of natural and inducible cyto-

toxic activities in mouse spleen cells. *Immunology* 1984; 51:727–733.

270. Schally AV: Oncological applications of somatostatin analogues. *Cancer Res* 1988; 48:6977–6985.

271. Schein RHM, et al: ICU survival of patients with the acquired immunodeficiency syndrome. *Crit Care Med* 1986; 14:1026–1027.

272. Schwarz K: Development and status of experimental work on factor 3 selenium. *Fed Proc* 1961; 20:666–673.

273. Schwarz K, Foltz CM: Selenium as an integral part of factor 3 against dietary necrotic liver degeneration. *J Am Chem Soc* 1957; 79:3292–3293.

274. Scuderi P, et al: Raised serum levels of tumor necrosis factor in parasitic infections. *Lancet* 1986; 2:1364–1365.

275. Sharer LR: AIDS virus and the brain. *West J Med* 1987; 146:88–90.

276. Sharer LR, et al: Pathologic features of AIDS encephalopathy in children: Evidence for LAV/HTLV-III infection of brain. *Hum Pathol* 1986; 17:271–284.

277. Sheldon GF: Septic complications of total parenteral nutrition. *Surgery* 1976; 132:214–218.

278. Shepherd JJ, et al: Regression of liver metastases in patients with gastrin-secreting tumor treated with SMS 201-995. *Lancet* 1986; 2:574.

279. Shike M, et al: Copper metabolism and requirements in total parenteral nutrition. *Gastroenterology* 1981; 81:290–297.

280. Shizgal HM, Forse RA: Protein and calorie requirements with total parenteral nutrition. *Ann Surg* 1980; 192:562–569.

281. Shoemaker JD, Millard MC, Johnson PB: Zinc in human immunodeficiency virus infection (letter). *JAMA* 1988 260:1881.

282. Siegler M, Weisbard AJ: Against the emerging stream: should fluids and nutritional support be discontinued? *Arch Intern Med* 1985; 145:129–131.

283. Silk DBA, et al: Uses of a peptide rather than free amino acid nitrogen source in chemically defined elemental diets. *JPEN* 1980; 4:548.

284. Sirisinha S, Suskind RM, Edelman R: Secretory and serum IgA in children with protein-caloric malnutrition. *Pediatrics* 1975; 55:166–170.

285. Sloper KS, et al: Chronic malabsorption due to cryptosporidiosis in a child with immunoglobulin deficiency. *Gut* 1982; 23:80–82.

286. Smith PD, Janoff EN: Infectious diarrhea in human immunodeficiency virus infection. *Gastro Clin North Am* 1988; 17:587–598.

287. Snider WD, et al: Neurological complications of acquired immune deficiency syndrome: Analysis of 50 patients. *Ann Neurol* 1983; 14:403–418.

288. Sobrado J, et al: The effect of lipid emulsions on reticuloendothelial system function in the injured animal. *JPEN* 1985; 9:559.

289. Souba WW: Glutamine metabolism in catabolic states: Role of the intestinal tract. Thesis, Harvard School of Public Health, Department of Nutritional Biochemistry, June 1984.

290. Souba WW: Interorgan ammonia metabolism in health and disease: A surgeon's view. *JPEN* 1987; 11:569–579.

291. Souba WW, Wilmore DW: Gut-liver interaction during accelerated gluconeogenesis. *Arch Surg* 1985; 120:66–70.

292. Souba WW, Wilmore DW: Postoperative alteration of arteriovenous exchange of amino acids across the gastrointestinal tract. *Surgery* 1983; 94:342–350.

293. Souba WW, Scott TE, Wilmore DW: Effect of glucocorticoids on glutamine metabolism in visceral organs. *Metabolism* 1985; 34:450.

294. Souba WW, Scott TA and Wilmore DW: Intestinal consumption of intravenously administered fuels. *JPEN* 1985; 9:18–22.

295. Souba WW, et al: Glutamine metabolism by the intestinal tract. *JPEN* 1985; 9:608–617.

296. Souba WW, et al: Glucocorticoids alter amino acid metabolism in visceral organs. *Surg Forum* 1983; 34:74.

297. Souba WW, et al: Interorgan glutamine metabolism in the tumor-bearing rat. *J Surg Res* 1988; 44:720–726.

298. Souba WW, et al: Postoperative alterations in interorgan glutamine exchange in enterectomized dogs. *J Surg Res* 1987; 42:117–125.

299. Spiller RC, Silk DBA: Malabsorption, in Kinney J, Jeejeebhoy K, Hill G, et al (eds): *Nutrition and Metabolism in Patient Care,* Philadelphia: WB Saunders Co/ Harcourt Brace Jovanovich, 1988, p 281.

300. Steinbrook R, Lo B: Artificial feeding—solid ground, not a slippery slope. *N Engl J Med* 1988; 318:286–290.

301. Steinbrook R, Lo B: Decision making for incompetent patients by designated proxy: California's new law. *N Engl J Med* 1984; 310:1598–1601.

302. Steinbrook R, et al: Preferences of homosexual men with AIDS for life-sustaining treatment. *N Engl J Med* 1986; 314:457–460.

303. Stemmermann GN, et al: Cryptosporidiosis: Report of a fatal case complicated by disseminated toxoplasmosis. *Am J Med* 1980; 69:637–642.

304. Stockmann F, et al: Long-term treatment of patients with endocrine gastrointestinal tumors with the somatostatin analogue SMS 201-995. *Scand J Gastroenterology* 1986; 21(suppl 119):230–237.

305. Stover DE, et al: Spectrum of pulmonary diseases associated with the acquired immunodeficiency syndrome. *Am J Med* 1985; 78:429–437.

306. Strom RL, Gruminger RP: AIDS with *Mycobacterium avium*-intracellular lesions resembling those of Whipple's disease (letter). *N Engl J Med* 1983; 309:1323.

307. Sundram CJ: Informed consent for major medical treatment of mentally disabled people. *N Engl J Med* 1988; 318:23–26.

308. Tanaka J, Fujiwara H, Torisu M: Vitamin E and immune response: Enhancement of helper T-cell activity by dietary supplementation of Vitamin E in mice. *Immunology* 1979; 38:727–734.

309. Tashiro T, et al: The effect of fat emulsion on essential fatty acid deficiency during intravenous hyperalimentation in pediatric patients. *J Pediatr Surg* 1975; 10:203–213.

310. Taub B: The nutritional implications of AIDS. *Environ Nutr* 1983; pp. 6:1–2.

311. Teppo AM, Maury CPJ: Radioimmunoassay of tumor necrosis factor in serum. *Clin Chem* 1987; 33:2024–2027.

312. Thompson CD, Robinson MF: Selenium in human health and disease with emphasis on those aspects peculiar to New Zealand. *Am J Clin Nutr* 1980; 33:303–333.

313. Torti FM, et al: A macrophage factor inhibits adipocyte gene expression: An in vitro mode of cachexia. *Science* 1985; 229:867–869.

314. Tracey KJ, et al: Cachectin/TNF induces cachexia, anemia and inflammation. *J Exp Med* 1988; 167:1211–1227.

315. Travis SF, et al: Alterations of red-cell glycolytic interme-diates and oxygen transport as a consequence of hypophos-phatemia in patients receiving intravenous hyperalimenta-tion. *N Engl J Med* 1971; 285:763–768.

316. Tzipori S, et al: Vomiting and diarrhea associated with cryptosporidial infection. *N Engl J Med* 1980; 303:818.

317. Update: Acquired immunodeficiency syndrome; United States. *MMWR* 1984; 32:688–691.

318. Van Rij AM, et al: Selenium supplementation in total par-enteral nutrition. *JPEN* 1981; 5:120–124.

319. Van Rij AM, et al: Selenium deficiency in total parenteral nutrition. *Am J Clin Nutr* 1979; 32:2076–2085.

320. Van Buren CT: *Nutrition* 1990; 6:105–106.

321. Van Buren, et al: The importance of lymphocyte migration patterns in experimental organ transplantation. *Transplanta-tion* 1986; 40:1–8.

322. Verschoor L, et al: On the use of a new somatostatin ana-logue in the treatment of hypoglycemia in patients with insulinoma. *Clin Endocrinol* 1986; 25:555–560.

323. Vinik A, Moattari AR: Use of somatostatin analogue in management of carcinoid syndrome. *Dig Dis Sci* 1989; 34:14S–27S.

324. Vinik A, et al: Somatostatin analogue (SMS 201-995) in the management of gastroenteropancreatic tumors and diar-rhea symptoms. *Am J Med* 1986; 81(suppl 6B):23–40.

325. Visek WJ: Arginine needs, physiological state and usual diets: A reevaluation. *J Nutr* 1986; 116:36–46.

326. Von Meyenfeldt MM, et al: TPN catheter sepsis: Lack of effect of subcutaneous tunnelling of PVC catheters on sep-sis rate. *JPEN* 1980; 4:514–517.

327. Wachter RM, et al: Intensive care of patients with acquired immunodeficiency syndrome. *Am Rev Respir Dis* 1986; 134:891–898.

328. Wanger SH, et al: The physician's responsibility toward hopelessly ill patients. *N Engl J Med* 1989; 320:844–849.

329. Watson RR: Nutrition and immunity. *J Dent Child* 1981; 48:443–446.

330. Weinberg DS, Murray HW: Coping with AIDS. The spe-cial problems of New York City. *N Engl J Med* 1987; 317:1469–1472.

331. Weinstein L, et al: Intestinal cryptosporidiosis complicated

by disseminated cytomegalovirus infection. *Gastroenterology* 1981; 81:584–591.

332. Weir JA: Trace elements of metalloenzymes. *Natl Intravenous Ther Assn,* 1981; 4:267–269.

333. Weisberg HF: Osmotic pressure of the serum proteins. *Ann Clin Lab Sci* 1978; 8:155–164.

334. Wharton JM, et al: Trimethoprim-sulfamethoxazole or pentamidine for *Pneumocystis carinii* pneumonia in the acquired immunodeficiency syndrome. *Ann Intern Med,* 1986; 105:37–44.

335. Whiteside ME, et al: Enteric coccidiosis among patients with the acquired immunodeficiency syndrome. *Am J Trop Med Hyg* 1984; 33:1065–1072.

336. WHO Expert Committee Report: Trace elements in human nutrition. *WHO Tech Rep Ser* 1973; 532:25, 65.

337. Wiley CA, et al: Cellular localization of human immunodeficiency virus infection within the brains of acquired immune deficiency syndrome patients. *Proc Natl Acad Sci USA* 1986; 83:7089–7093.

338. Wintrobe MM, et al: *Clinical Hematology.* Philadelphia: Lea & Febiger, 1974.

339. Wolfe RR, et al: Investigation of factors determining the optimal glucose infusion rate in total parenteral nutrition. *Metabolism* 1980; 29:892.

340. Wolman SL, et al: Zinc in total parenteral nutrition: Requirements and metabolic effects. *Gastroenterology* 1979; 76:458–467.

341. Wood SM, et al: Treatment of patients with pancreatic endocrine tumors using a new long-acting somatostatin analogue. Symptomatic and peptide responses. *Gut* 1985; 26:438–444.

342. Xhen XS, et al: Studies on the relations of selenium and Keshan disease. *Biol Trace Elements Res* 1980; 2:91–107.

343. Young VR: Selenium: A case for its essentiality in man. *N Engl J Med* 1981; 34:1228–1230.

344. Zagoren AJ, et al: Colloid osmotic pressure: Sensitive predictor of enteral feeding tolerance. *J Am Coll Nutr* 1984; 4:260.

KEY RECOMMENDED READINGS

For a list of key recommended readings for Chapter 4, see Appendix 2, pp. 289 and 290.

SELF-ASSESSMENT QUESTIONS

Directions. Select the best response to each of the questions or statements below and enter the corresponding letter in the space provided.

( ) 1. Patients with AIDS often have significant _____ depletion.
   A. Potassium
   B. Body fat
   C. Intracellular water volume
   D. Serum protein
   E. All of the above

see p. 185

( ) 2. Patients with AIDS have an average weight loss of 16% from their preillness usual weight prior to death.
   A. True
   B. False

see p. 185

( ) 3. Malnutrition results in all of the following, **except:**
   A. Reduction in the total number of T-lymphocytes, helper, and suppressor cells
   B. Impaired cell-mediated and secretory immunity
   C. Improved phagocyte activity
   D. Decreased killer cell activity

see p. 185

( ) 4. Mineral, trace metal, and vitamin deficiencies adversely affect the PWA's:
   A. Immune function
   B. Recovery from secondary infection
   C. Response to chemotherapy
   D. All of the above

see p. 186

( ) 5. The following factors should be considered when formulating a nutritional therapy regimen for PWAs: (1) epidemiologic and economic data, (2) psychosocial status, (3) etiologies for gut dysfunction, (4) nutrient requirements, (5) therapeutic goal, (6) treatment options, (7) types of diets, and (8) specific therapeutic regimens.

A. True
B. False

see p. 186

( ) 6. According to the World Health Organization, 15 to 20 million people worldwide will be HIV-positive by the year 2000.

A. True
B. False

see p. 187

( ) 7. AIDS-related medical costs (excluding nutritional therapy) for the 270,000 U.S. AIDS cases diagnosed between 1981 and the end of 1991 are projected to be $22 billion.

A. True
B. False

see p. 187

( ) 8. The central nervous system and psychologic effects of an HIV infection can adversely affect the PWA's:

A. Daily activities
B. Response to medical therapy
C. Nutrient intake
D. All of the above

see p. 188

( ) 9. PWAs with oral thrush, ulcers, and mucosites may experience:

A. Progressive weight loss
B. Burning sensation or dysphagia with food ingestion
C. A only
D. A and B

see p. 192

( ) 10. Patients with an intestinal HIV infection often have massive diarrhea and subsequently develop:

A. Electrolyte imbalance

B. Dehydration

C. Trace metal deficiencies

see p. 193

( ) 11. PWAs with a CMV intestinal infection may have gastrointestinal symptoms similar to a patient with:

A. Inflammatory bowel disease

B. Intestinal tuberculosis

C. A volvulus

D. None of the above

see p. 193

( ) 12. Which of the following bacterial infections occur in PWAs?

A. *Shigella*

B. *Mycobacterium avium-intracellulare*

C. *Campylobacter*

D. *All of the above*

see p. 193

( ) 13. PWAs with a *Cryptosporidium* infection of the gut often develop severe, profuse, secretory diarrhea which is refractory to chemo and antidiarrheal therapy. Unless successfully treated, these patients rapidly:

A. Become dehydrated

B. Develop electrolyte and trace metal deficiencies

C. Become malnourished

D. All of the above

see p. 193

( ) 14. Kaposi's sarcoma, the most common alimentary tract tumor found in PWAs, may cause which of the following:

A. Oral pain

B. Dysphagia

C. Intractable diarrhea

    D. Incomplete or complete bowel obstruction

    E. All of the above

see p. 193

( ) 15. Protein-calorie malnutrition is the most common type of malnutrition occurring among PWAs.

    A. True

    B. False

see p. 195

( ) 16. An HIV infection may cause which of the following:

    A. Villous destruction and altered gut function

    B. Decreased absorptive surface in the gut

    C. Impaired digestion

    D. All of the above

see p. 195

( ) 17. All of the following may occur during sepsis, **except:**

    A. Increased serum total protein

    B. Reduction in muscle mass

    C. Hypoalbuminemia

    D. Negative nitrogen balance

see p. 196

( ) 18. Instead of sequentially using glucose, fat, and finally amino acids, as in a milder state of starvation, energy production in the septic state becomes progressively protein based.

    A. True

    B. False

see p. 196

( ) 19. PWAs suffering from protein-calorie malnutrition have _____.

    A. Reduced or absent cutaneous hypersensitivity response to common microbial antigens

    B. Decreased number of thymus-dependent T-lymphocytes

    C. Reduced T-4 helper cells

    D. Reduced T-8 cytotoxic, suppressor cells.

    E. All of the above.

see p. 197

( ) 20. All of the following statements are true regarding glutamine, **except:**

A. Most abundant amino acid in both whole blood and the intracellular free amino acid pool

B. Major oxidative substrate for the small intestine

C. Concentration in whole blood and skeletal muscle increases markedly following injury or during catabolic disease states.

D. Glutamine metabolism by the intestine generates alanine.

see p. 198

( ) 21. Patients with AIDS should receive enteral and parenteral diets fortified with _____ to maintain the integrity of the small bowel mucosa and to enhance the absorption of nutrients.

A. Omega-6 fats

B. Long-chain triglycerides

C. Glutamine

D. Lactulose

see p. 198

( ) 22. All of the following statements are true regarding arginine, **except:**

A. Semi-essential amino acid

B. Patients receiving arginine-supplemented enteral diets had significant enhancement in their T-lymphocyte activation to concanavalin A and phytohemagglutinin and an increase in mean CD4 phenotype.

C. The endogenous synthesis of arginine is closely linked with the urea cycle enzymes of both the liver and kidney.

D. Supplemental arginine has been shown to reduce immunocompetence in patients whose cellular immunity was impaired by the metabolic status of illness and surgery

see p. 199

( ) 23. T-lymphocytes and intestinal epithelial cells appear to lack the ability to synthesize nucleotides.

    A. True
    B. False

see p. 202

( ) 24. Nucleotide-free diets have been reported to:

    A. Decrease delayed hypersensitivity responses
    B. Decrease resistance to infection
    C. Decrease IL-2 production
    D. All of the above

see p. 204

( ) 25. Selenium deficiency has been associated with which of the following?

    A. Fungal infection
    B. Increased risk of neoplastic disease
    C. Congestive heart failure
    D. All of the above

see p. 204

( ) 26. A zinc deficiency in non-AIDS patients with primary hypogammaglobulinemia is associated with an impaired proliferative response to mitogens and depressed T-killer cell activity.

    A. True
    B. False

see p. 205

( ) 27. A copper deficiency results in all of the following, **except:**

    A. Increased incidence of infection
    B. Depressed reticuloendothelial cell function
    C. Increased microbial activity of the granulocytes
    D. Neurologic dysfunction

see p. 205

( ) 28. An iron deficiency results in all of the following, **except:**

    A. Impaired lymphocyte response to mitogens

B. Increased neutrophil bactericidal capacity
C. Fatigue
D. Palpitations

see p. 205

( ) 29. Which of the following statements regarding polyunsaturated fatty acids (PUFAs) are true?

A. Cell-to-cell communication may be modulated by altering the dietary PUFAs' composition.
B. PUFAs are classified into two major families: omega-6 and omega-3 PUFAs.
C. Alpha linolenic acid (omega-3 PUFAs) is present in linseed, canola, walnut, and soybean oils.
D. Cold water fish are a rich source of omega-3 PUFAs.
E. All of the above.

see p. 206

( ) 30. In individuals with primary pernicious anemia, the lymphocyte response to mitogens is improved and neutrophilic, phagocytic, and bacterial capacity are enhanced.

A. True
B. False

see p. 210

( ) 31. A pyridoxine (vitamin B₆) deficiency results in depressed cellular and humoral immunity.

A. True
B. False

see p. 210

( ) 32. A vitamin A deficiency results in:

A. Depletion of thymic lymphocytes
B. Depressed lymphocyte response to various mitogens
C. Impaired secretory IgA production and T-cell function
D. All of the above

see p. 210

( ) 33. All PWAs considered for nutritional therapy must satisfy the following screening criteria: (1) a recent unintentional 10% decrease in the their reference weight or (2) at least a 20-lb weight loss compared to their usual weight.

    A. True
    B. False

see p. 211

( ) 34. A nutritional assessment should include which of the following?

    A. Evaluation of key nutritional indices
    B. A 24-hr nitrogen balance determination
    C. Assessment of gastrointestinal function
    D. Estimate of the patient's daily caloric and protein requirements
    E. All of the above

see p. 212

( ) 35. Which of the following is the most important nutritional index to consider prior to initiating nutritional therapy?

    A. Somatic protein reserve
    B. Visceral protein reserve
    C. Fat reserve
    D. 24-hr nitrogen balance

see p. 212

( ) 36. Malnourished PWAs require _____ kcal/kg/day to prevent further weight loss and to maintain nutritional homeostasis.

    A. 20–25
    B. 30–35
    C. 35–40
    D. 40–45

see p. 213

( ) 37. Malnourished PWAs require _____ g of protein/kg/day to prevent further weight loss and to maintain nutritional homeostasis.

    A. 0.4–0.8

B. 0.8–1.5
C. 1.5–2.0
D. 2.0–2.5

see p. 214

( ) 38. An ideal enteral diet for PWAs should contain all of the following, **except:**

A. Low molecular weight (MW) proteins (MW <500 daltons) in the form of either free amino acids or polypeptides
B. Glutamine (>10% of the total amino acid content)
C. Adequate amounts of electrolytes, minerals, and trace metals, including selenium, chromium, and molybdenum.
D. Large amount of fat (>20% of the total calories) and lactose

see p. 216

( ) 39. A liter of peripheral parenteral nutrition (PPN) solution for PWAs should contain which of the following?

A. $D_{20}W$ 500 cc
B. Amino acids 10% 500 cc
C. Electrolytes, vitamins, minerals, and trace metals, including selenium, chromium, and molybdenum
D. All of the above

see p. 226

( ) 40. A liter of total parenteral nutrition (TPN) solution for PWAs should contain which of the following?

A. $D_{60}W$ 500 cc
B. Amino acids 10% 500 cc
C. Electrolytes, vitamins, minerals, and trace metals, including selenium, chromium, and molybdenum
D. All of the above

see p. 227

Directions. Match statements #41–60 with the appropriate diet or pharmacologic agent listed below and enter the corresponding letter in the space provided. NOTE: The diets and pharmacologic agents may be used *more* than once.

A. Vivonex T.E.N.
B. Albumin
C. Carnation Instant Breakfast
D. Compleat Modified Formula
E. Megace
F. Impact
G. TPN
H. Hespan
I. Resource
J. Sandostatin
K. PPN
L. Reabilan HN
M. ProcalAmine

( ) 41. Excellent synthetic plasma expander used to enhance enteral diet tolerance by increasing the patient's serum colloid osmotic pressure (COP) and bowel wall oncotic pressure (BWOP). see p. 242

( ) 42. "Pre-mixed" peripheral parenteral nutrition (PPN) solution which derives its calories from glycerol.
see p. 226

( ) 43. Contains arginine, nucleotides, and omega-3 PUFAs and may be helpful in improving the PWA's nutritional status and overall immunocompetence.
see p. 223

( ) 44. Contains the highest percentage of low molecular weight (MW <1,000 D) polypeptides.
see p. 224

( ) 45. A "mixed," short-term (<10 days) method of parenteral nutrition therapy for PWAs who cannot tolerate an oral or nasointestinal enteral diet and require bowel rest. see p. 226

( ) 46. Andrassy formula. see p. 241

( ) 47. Pure amino acid diet containing 100% amino acids (MW <500 D), adequate electrolytes, minerals, vitamins, trace metals (including selenium, chromium, and molybdenum), glutamine, <3% fat, and branchial chain amino acids. see p. 217

( ) 48. Preferred nasointestinal enteral diet for PWAs with a "nonspecific" or "enteropathic" enteropathy.
see p. 239

( ) 49. Approved by the FDA as a breast and endometrial antineoplastic agent but *not* as an appetite stimulant.
see p. 238

( ) 50. Synthetic octapeptide which appears to be very effective in treating AIDS-related diarrhea.
see p. 228

( ) 51. Prolonged therapy (>3 months) is very controversial both ethically and economically.
see p. 230

( ) 52. Preferred oral food supplement for malnourished PWAs with normal gut function.
see p. 217

( ) 53. Blenderized, meat-based, intact protein enteral diet used to treat PWAs with normal gut function or patients with enteral diet induced diarrhea.
see p. 222

( ) 54. Mixed with vitamin D whole milk and used as an alternative oral food supplement for malnourished PWAs with normal gut function.
see p. 222

( ) 55. Combined with Sandostatin to treat malnourished PWAs requiring nutritional therapy >10 days, <3 months.
see p. 230

( ) 56. Alternate, intact protein, modular, oral food supplement (does not require reconstitution with whole vitamin D milk) used to treat PWAs with a "nonspecific" or "enteropathic" enteropathy. (See "Intact Protein . . . Supplements.")
see p. 221

( ) 57. Contraindicated in PWAs with CNS pathology or emotional instability.

see p. 230

( ) 58. Specific criteria must be satisfied prior to initiating therapy.

see p. 230

( ) 59. National shortage.

see p. 241

( ) 60. No solution wastage if the therapy is terminated.

see p. 226

APPENDIX 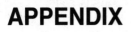 1

SELF-ASSESSMENT ANSWERS

CHAPTER 1

1. **C**	14. **A**	27. **D**	39. **A**
2. **C**	15. **B**	28. **B**	40. **A**
3. **C**	16. **A**	29. **A**	41. **A**
4. **B**	17. **C**	30. **D**	42. **A**
5. **D**	18. **C**	31. **B**	43. **A**
6. **D**	19. **A**	32. **B**	44. **C**
7. **B**	20. **B**	33. **D**	45. **D**
8. **B**	21. **A**	34. **B**	46. **A**
9. **D**	22. **D**	35. **A**	47. **A**
10. **E**	23. **A**	36. **D**	48. **C**
11. **C**	24. **D**	37. **B**	49. **A**
12. **C**	25. **D**	38. **B**	50. **C**
13. **B**	26. **D**		

CHAPTER 2

1. **C**	14. **A**	27. **D**	39. **K**
2. **D**	15. **B**	28. **D**	40. **H**
3. **A**	16. **D**	29. **D**	41. **A**
4. **A**	17. **C**	30. **A**	42. **H**
5. **A**	18. **A**	31. **L**	43. **B**

6.	**E**	19.	**C**	32.	**I**	44.	**F**
7.	**C**	20.	**B**	33.	**F**	45.	**I**
8.	**A**	21.	**B**	34.	**E**	46.	**J**
9.	**D**	22.	**B**	35.	**J**	47.	**G**
10.	**D**	23.	**A**	36.	**G**	48.	**D**
11.	**B**	24.	**A**	37.	**D**	49.	**I**
12.	**A**	25.	**A**	38.	**C**	50.	**L**
13.	**A**	26.	**D**				

CHAPTER 3

1.	**A**	14.	**B**	27.	**D**	39.	**A**
2.	**A**	15.	**B**	28.	**B**	40.	**A**
3.	**D**	16.	**D**	29.	**D**	41.	**A**
4.	**E**	17.	**B**	30.	**D**	42.	**A**
5.	**D**	18.	**C**	31.	**C**	43.	**A**
6.	**A**	19.	**A**	32.	**A**	44.	**A**
7.	**C**	20.	**D**	33.	**C**	45.	**C**
8.	**B**	21.	**A**	34.	**A**	46.	**D**
9.	**D**	22.	**B**	35.	**D**	47.	**A**
10.	**B**	23.	**B**	36.	**A**	48.	**A**
11.	**A**	24.	**D**	37.	**A**	49.	**D**

| 12. | E | 25. | D | 38. | B | 50. | B |
| 13. | C | 26. | A | | | | |

CHAPTER 4

1.	E	16.	D	31.	B	46.	B
2.	A	17.	A	32.	D	47.	A
3.	C	18.	A	33.	A	48.	A
4.	D	19.	E	34.	E	49.	E
5.	A	20.	C	35.	B	50.	J
6.	A	21.	C	36.	D	51.	G
7.	A	22.	D	37.	D	52.	A
8.	D	23.	A	38.	D	53.	D
9.	D	24.	D	39.	D	54.	C
10.	D	25.	D	40.	D	55.	G
11.	A	26.	A	41.	H	56.	I
12.	D	27.	C	42.	M	57.	G
13.	D	28.	B	43.	F	58.	G
14.	E	29.	E	44.	L	59.	B
15.	A	30.	B	45.	K	60.	M

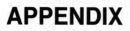# APPENDIX

2

KEY RECOMMENDED READINGS

CHAPTER 1

Askanazi J, et al: Nutritional care of the trauma patient. *Surg Gynecol Obstet* 1983; 157:585–597.

Bower RH: Nutritional and metabolic support of critically ill patients. *JPEN J Parenter Enteral Nutr* 1990; 14(suppl):257S–259S.

Cerra FB: How nutrition intervention changes what getting sick means. *JPEN J Parenter Enteral Nutr* 1990; 14(suppl):164S–169S.

Christou N: Perioperative nutritional support: Immunologic defects. *JPEN J Parenter Enteral Nutr* 1990; 14(suppl):186S–192S.

Curreri WP: Metabolic response to thermal injury and its nutritional support. *Cutis* 1978, 22;501.

Detsky AS, et al: Predicting nutrition-associated complications for patients undergoing gastrointestinal surgery. *JPEN* 1987; 11:440–446.

Grant J: Nutritional assessment in clinical practice. *Nutr Clin Prac* 1986; 1:3–11.

Hickey MS: Enteral and parenteral nutrition, in Katzung BG (ed): *Clinical Manual of Drug Therapy*. San Mateo, Calif, Appleton and Lange, 1991, 387–402.

Hickey MS: Nutrition, in Trunkey DD, Lewis FR (eds): *Current Therapy of Trauma,* ed 3. Philadelphia; BC Decker, 1991, pp 78–94.

Jeejeebhoy KN, et al: Assessment of nutritional status. *JPEN J Parenter Enteral Nutr* 1990; 14(suppl):193S–196S.

Kinney JM, et al: Indirect calorimetry in malnutrition: Nutritional assessment or therapeutic reference? *JPEN* 1987; 11:(suppl):905–995.

Lazlo JK, et al: Clinical application of the metabolic cart to the delivery of total parenteral nutrition. *Crit Care Med* 1990; 18:1320–1327.

CHAPTER 2

Askanazi J, et al: Nutrition and the respiratory system. *Crit Care Med* 1982; 10:163–172.

American Society for Parenteral and Enteral Nutrition, Board of Directors. Guidelines for the use of enteral nutrition in adult patients. *JPEN J Parenter Enteral Nutr* 1987; 11:435–439.

Brinson RR, et al. Intestinal absorption of peptide enteral formulas in hypoproteinemic (volume expanded) rats: A paired analysis. *Crit Care Med* 1989; 17:657–660.

Daly JM, et al: Dietary protein prevents bacterial translocation from the gut. *JPEN* 1991; 15(suppl):295.

Kinsella JE: Lipids, membrane receptors, and enzymes: Effects of dietary fatty acids. *JPEN,* Vol. 14, No. 5, *J Parenter Enteral Nutr* 1990; 14(suppl):200s–217s.

Kirk SJ, Barbul A: Role of arginine in trauma, sepsis, and immunity. *JPEN, J Parenter Enteral Nutr* 1990; 14(suppl):226s–229s.

Fischer JE: Branched-chain-enriched amino acid solutions in patients with liver failure: An early example of nutritional pharmacology. *JPEN J Parenter Enteral Nutr* 1990; 14(suppl):249s–256s.

Foley EF, et al: Albumin supplementation in the critically ill patient. *Arch Surg* 1990; 125:739–742.

Good RA, Lorenz E: Influence of energy levels and trace metals on health and life span. *JPEN, J Parenter Enteral Nutr* 1990; 14(suppl):230S–236S.

Hickey MS: Enteral and parenteral nutrition, in Katzung BG(ed): *Clinical Manual of Drug Therapy.* San Mateo, Calif: Appleton and Lange, 1991, pp 387–402.

Hickey MS: Nutrition, in: Trunkey DD, Lewis FR (eds): *Current Therapy of Trauma,* ed 3. Philadelphia, BC Decker, 1991, pp 78–94.

Moore FA, et al: TEN vs TPN following major abdominal trauma—reduced morbidity. *J Trauma* 1989; 29:916–923.

Souba WW, et al: Glutamine nutrition: Theoretical considerations and therapeutic impact. *JPEN J Parenter Enteral Nutr* 1990; 14(suppl):237S–243S.

CHAPTER 3

American Society for Parenteral and Enteral Nutrition, Board of Directors. Guidelines for the use of home total parenteral nutrition. *JPEN J Parenter Enteral Nutr* 1987; 11:342–344.

American Society for Parenteral and Enteral Nutrition, Board of Directors. Guidelines for the use of total parenteral nutrition in the hospitalized adult patient. *JPEN J Parenter Enteral Nutr* 1986; 10:441–445.

Conly JM, et al: A propsective, randomized study comparing transparent and dry gauze dressings for central venous catheters. *J Infect Dis* 1989; 159:310–319.

Coppa GF, et al: Air embolism: A lethal but preventable complication of subclavian vein catheterization. *JPEN J Parenter Enteral Nutr* Vol. 5, 1981; 5:166–168.

Fischer JE: Nutritional support. *Natl Intravenous Ther Assoc* 1981; 4:431–435.

Freund H, et al: Comparative study of parenteral nutrition in renal failure using essential and non-essential amino acid containing solutions. *Surg Gynecol Obstet* 1980; 151:652–656.

Hickey MS: Enteral and parenteral nutrition, in Katzung BG (ed): *Clinical Manual of Drug Therapy.* San Mateo, Calif: Appleton and Lange, 1991, pp 387–402.

Hickey MS: Nutrition, in Trunkey DD, Lewis FR (eds): *Current Therapy of Trauma,* ed 3. Philadelphia, BC Decker, 1991, pp 78–94.

McCarthy MC, et al: Prospective evaluation of single and triple lumen catheters in total parenteral nutrition. *JPEN J Parenter Enteral Nutr* 1987; 11:259–262.

Silberman H: The safety and efficacy of a lipid-based system of parenteral nutrition in acute pancreatitis. *Gastroenterology* 1982; 77:494–497.

Wagman LD, et al: The effect of acute discontinuance of total parenteral nutrition. *Ann Surg* 1986; 204:524–529.

Wolk R: Metabolic complications and deficiencies of parenteral nutrition. *Compr Ther* 1985; 11:67–75.

CHAPTER 4

American Society for Parenteral and Enteral Nutrition. 12th Clinical Congress: Care and management of AIDS patients. Las Vegas, Nev, January 17, 1988.

Cello JP, et al: Controlled clinical trial of octreotide for refractory AIDS-associated diarrhea. Abstract 163 presented at the American Digestive Week Meeting, San Antonio, Tex, May 1990.

Chlebowski RT, et al: Nutritional status, gastrointestinal dysfunction, and survival in patients with AIDS. *Am J Gastroenterol* 1989; 84:1288–1293.

Garcia ME, et al: The acquired immune deficiency syndrome: Nutritional complications and assessment of body weight status. *Nutr Clin Prac* 1987; 21:108–111.

Hickey MS: Nutritional support of patients with AIDS. *Surg Clin North Am* 1991; 71:645–664.

Hickey MS, Weaver KE: Nutritional management of patients with ARC or AIDS. *Gastroenterol Clin North Am* 1988; 17:545–561.

Kotler DP: Diarrhea in AIDS-diagnosis and management. *Res Staff Phys* 1987; 33:30–41.

Kotler DP, et al: Effect of home total parenteral nutrition on body composition in patients with acquired immunodeficiency syndrome. *JPEN J Parenter Enteral Nutr* 1990; 5:454–458.

Kotler DP, et al: Magnitude of body-cell-mass depletion and the timing of death from wasting in AIDS. *Am J Clin Nutr* 1989; 50:444–447.

McCorkindale C, et al: Nutritional status of HIV-infected patients during the early disease stages. *J Am Dietetic Assn,* 1990; 90:1236–1241.

Robinson EN, Fuegel R: SMS 201–295, a Somatostatin analogue and diarrhea in the acquired immunodeficiency syndrome (AIDS). *Ann Intern Med,* 1988; 109:680–681.

Sax HC: Practicalities of lipids: ICU patient, autoimmune disease, and vascular disease. *JPEN J Parenter Enteral Nutr* 1990; 14(Suppl):223S–225S.

INDEX